# Choices for the Choiceless

## "The Lost Sheep"

by

Nanette Phillips

*AuthorHouse™*
*1663 Liberty Drive*
*Bloomington, IN 47403*
*www.authorhouse.com*
*Phone: 833-262-8899*

*The information contained in this book is not intended to treat any illness.*

*Published by AuthorHouse 06/17/2021*

*ISBN: 978-1-4184-4817-2 (sc)*

*Print information available on the last page.*

*I DEDICATE THIS BOOK TO MANY PEOPLE BUT WILL ONLY BE ABLE TO MENTION A FEW. THEY ARE ALL ROLE MODELS IN THEIR OWN RIGHT. SOME WHOM I KNOW AND SOME I HAVE NEVER MET, BUT ALL AN INSPIRING FORCE FOR ME TO CREATE, DILIGENTLY SUFFICE, AND ULTIMATELY COMPLETE THIS LITERARY WORK.*

*TO MY MOTHER WHO HAS INSPIRED ME TO WRITE THIS BOOK BY HER WILL TO NEVER GIVE UP EVEN THROUGH TIMES OF TOTAL SICKNESS AND DESPAIR, SHE IS THE PERSONIFICATION OF TRUE STRENGTH.*

*TO MY SON, WHO SUPPORTED ME AND IS A CONSTANT REMINDER THAT LOVE FOR YOUR FAMILY AND FELLOW MAN IS THE MOST IMPORTANT PART OF LIFE.*

*TO MY GRANDMOTHER, ADDIE, WHOM I NEVER MET BUT THROUGH MY MOTHER EXISTED IN MY HEART DAILY AND BECAME A PROFOUND ROLE MODEL AND POSITIVE INFLUENCE IN MY LIFE.*

*TO OTHER FAMILY MEMBERS, AND FRIENDS WHO UNKNOWINGLY THROUGH THEIR ATTENTIVE AND OFTEN TIMES NOT SO ATTENTIVE EARS WHOM WITHOUT I AM NOT.*

ΔΦΦΦΦΦΦΦΦΦΦΦΦΦΔ

*THE STRONGEST PRINCIPLE OF GROWTH LIES IN HUMAN CHOICE.*
*--------GEORGE ELIOT-------*

Preface

What are you looking for the answer is behind you!

So we carry a lot of excess baggage physically as well mentally, and blame others for our mistakes as we run from our previous mistakes and make even more mistakes, all the while just continuing the vicious circle. In order for the lost to find their way back in the right direction, they must take a look behind in the past, not staying or even dwelling in it, but attempting to evaluate the choices we are making and make the right change. Never wavering just pushing forward to reverse the unanswered past, while leaving what if's behind.

For all of us are a product of previously made choices, and now must choose if we want to continue on just merely existing with little or no mental thought process, or whether the lost sheep will evaluate and educate our selves to the most often distance and hidden why's of these decisions. One gains knowledge by past experiences and education through reading the old as well as the new findings. Sometimes we find out answers to our what if's and why's, most often through reading. Maybe someone has been through what you are going through and their own self-help can in fact help others cope or avoid mistakes.

Moreover to address our unrelenting and impetuous mental state it quite often requires a change in our physical realm first, and there could not be a more significant statement than 'you are what you eat' as you will learn in this book.

This is a bittersweet story of a woman finding truth, while dealing with life's most difficult choices. Although I relish most of my childhood memories that help shape individuality, I share some very painful situations including alcoholism and a childhood molestation incident, which help exacerbate mostly disheartening adult relationship mistakes. Growing up impoverished and experiencing further setbacks such as teenage and even adult molestation, I still manage to breakthrough all the obstacles, and achieve a lifelong dream of acquiring a college education. Finally experiencing mental along with physical healing from some bad relationship choices, I made the ultimate choice that proved to be the most difficult yet fulfilling decision which encompassed caring for a disabled and infirmed parent. This leads to the conclusion that there is a profound cause and effect for all of life's favorable as well as unfavorable outcomes. Finally after reversing some of the debilitating effects of an aging parent for a few years, I find healing for myself in the process. Then very unexpectedly other debilitating health disasters started to occur, but I feel I still triumph through the hard times. By never wavering in my faith while ultimately concluding that I, like many others exhibit inadequate knowledge in today's fast pace and continually changing society. But by documenting my mother's care as well as my own self-care, and researching numerous supplements and their purposes I gained a sense of security. The security in knowing that long-term dietary principals or habits along with exercise, as well as a continuous essential cleansing program for the body may contribute to sustaining an overall healthy life. Not only do these principals contribute to a disease free life, but also a healthy mental state which results in lifelong success and an overall positive view of one's life even as one ages.

Quiet simply this book is about the trials of life, never giving up, and continuing to seek real life changing answers. Thereby, gaining knowledge from every trial of life through educating yourself, which is sometimes given freely or learned through missteps. In chronological order I share my life as well as documenting the regiment of care for an aging infirmed parent. It includes lots of knowledgeable and interesting reading for literally everyone. Finally, this book is ultimately a celebration of life and celebration of death when each are within their appropriate time, although more often than not we control and choose that appointed time inappropriately.

*Table of Contents:*

## Introduction: 'Quality of Life'

Today there are a lot of issues on the political agenda. Whether it may be abortion, human rights, welfare reform, or some other never ending debatable issue. There are plenty of hot topics and success stories in the news and competition to be the number one in whatever aspect of our busy and most cherished industry you may pleasure. Whether it is the number one magazine, the number one company in profits, or to be the number one show in television, but I would like to bring everyone's attention back a minute to real life issues and that is the question of life and the quality of it.

I do not have a political agenda or a desire to be a hot topic, nor can I say that I am striving to be number one in any sense of the word. But I am one who desires peace of mind. As my mind appears to be a bit cloudy at this point because only a few hours ago a baby was aborted by me, and I am finding it extremely difficult dealing with it as my mother lay anguished in a nursing home less than two miles away from me. Although writing appears to be rather difficult as well, it is the only avenue I have found to deal with this difficulty in my life right now. As I continue to ask myself what am I doing with my life, and what is my life's purpose?

*Asking God what would you have me do with my life? I feel such a sense of lost, as there must be something more than this misery. My life seems so out of control as I have no control over my emotions much less my actions, and certainly no control over my mother's condition. As the tears continuously flow, it seems like I will never have any comfort from this tragedy. I feel so helpless as I cry out to God to forgive me, and give to this lost sheep direction and wisdom.*

*My life may or may not be different than any other, but in one sense I do feel it could have been even worst. At least I am alive this day and able to write about my life experiences which I hope will be able to enlighten someone else, while attempting to heal my own seemingly doomed soul. Even if my healing does not occur this day, maybe it will be feasible in future days to come in my life.*

*Today, I am finding it very hard to hold back the tears of a sometimes harsh yet gratifying reality, and the reality is that I have a right to choose. A right to choose is a privilege as well as a cherished honor for every single American. After coming of age into a role of adulthood, I found I have the right to choose my whole position and lifestyle on many different issues and matters of great importance in life. I have the right to choose whether or not to attend a school of higher learning, and choose the profession of my choice. I have the right to attend trade school or make a living by just merely going out and finding any job, if I can find one. I have a right to choose where or even who I would like to live with, possibly alone or marry. Whether I may want to have a child or two or maybe none. Even whether or not to care for an aging parent or just give up living life to its fullest and just merely exist.*

*All these equitable rights are tremendous significant privileges, and should be honored and cherished by anyone who may have the right to choose from these abundant choices.*

*Although some of these decisions we may have control, most often previously made decisions of others may overshadow one's right to choose. We are born into circumstances and influences that are not our own. And as a result of previously made decisions by others we somehow become mirror image persuasions of the past, which echoes into our predestined futures if we choose to let it. These previously made choices most often are made before we are even born, and can adhere to either a positive or a negative existence. Eventually, depending on what these decisions encompass they can cast feelings of hopelessness over one's life, which could ultimately give rise to a possible negative destiny.*

*It is very difficult and often times improbable for those who have not been exposed to circumstances other than what is around them to be anything different from that exposure. For example, if all I have been exposed to is hopelessness or even a meager or rather negative existence, then one can safely assume I will be a person who does not have much hope. If your surrounding or influences are relatively negative, then you will probably lack all hope. The kind of hope that would encompass goals and dreams of a fulfilling a meaningful future existence filled with love, and contributing to a better happier life for yourself as well as others.*

*Hence, hopelessness breeds hopelessness unless one is exposed to situations of hope. Hope is the only way one can expect to impact and achieve a meaningful quality of life. This stems from a vital and positive environment. If you do not have any hope or some type of inspiration to challenge your current circumstances, then how can one understand or even know how to make a relatively stronger and more meaningful existence.*

*Hope stems not only from observing your current surroundings, but also from observing past influences. Are those influences good? Do they make you feel good about yourself and give you a sense of purpose or feeling of well being which breeds hope and a positive outlook for your future?  Do these influences cause you to think about your present circumstances and compel you to want to make your life different or rather better?*

*Perhaps these influences that are most prevalent in your life causes you to just merely want a change.  Not necessarily for the better, because no one has ever challenged your place in life. Moreover your future plans do not encompass a desire to succeed, nor do you want to accomplish any goals.  All you want is the change, you just want out of your current situation without examining all aspects of your choices.  You have never been challenged to think of long-term objectives.  Nor are you compelled or desire to make a difference in your life or anyone else's for that matter.  You may just merely want to control your own life without any meaningful direction.  Maybe you have never even thought or given any regard to any type of plan, now or for your future.  Perhaps no one even talked to you about your future plans and if someone were to ask, you would be in awe.  Leaving you in mere bliss and possible unconcern due to your lack of exposure to the subject.*

*We sometimes make choices in what I term choice-less circumstances, because we are forced to make decisions on situations that we did not have any previous control over. Entering into the world just as lost sheep without a shepherd longing for a purpose, a pass, and a reason to exist. We can further sometimes remain as lost sheep without proper guidance or role models.*

*I have found through my life experiences no matter if you are born wealthy, poor, or the status of your family background we all have some reasonable choices we have to make in life.  The important aspect in life is the fact that you are aware you have choices.  You are responsible for your life and you can make good choices rather than bad.  The key aspect of making a good choice is that someone, whether it is our parents or some other role model, has exposed us to life's choice of hope. I feel fortunate for being exposed to hope in my seemingly hopeless existence. But some of us must go pass our immediate role models and look to teachers, neighbors, or whomever we may be exposed too for that positive existence. We must realize that no matter who you are and where you are in life, if you are an adult and a child is exposed to you, you are in fact a role model. Whether or not you choose to even be a role model, you are either a positive or negative role model.*

*Today, as I care for my son as well as my incapacitated mother who lost the ability to walk and care for herself, and she recently lost the ability to talk and even feed herself; this day I consider it a privilege. Not only to be a role model but to able to assist my mother, because I know she would do it for another as she, a role model in her own right has already helped many in her lifetime. But I did not always materialize my compassion in this manner.*

*I further understand that by making the not so good judgment calls in my life, I gave rise to the level of compassion that has manifested in my life today. Although I have lacked in certain areas of making the proper choices, it is almost as though it was fate silently working. Although I respect people who are empowered to make their own logical choices, I further feel my choices empowered me in the sense that I would otherwise not be the person I am this day. Through all my so called regrettable choices I kept the faith, hope, and dreams that somehow became embedded deep within my heart from childhood which I never lost but rather eventually expounded into even greater heights and aspirations.*

*As I believe our forefathers of this great country sailed over with only a dream, with merely hope and faith of a religious freedom. There were not any over 500-acre farms, houses, not one big city, or any signs of any future existence and growth. But today I am sure they would not marvel at this great country from the Atlantic to Pacific and growth beyond their wildest imagination, because the religious few had the faith and believed. Hence faith is synonymous with dreams as the biblical definition suggests. Faith is substance of things hoped for and the evidence of things not yet seen; faith is in fact one man's dream. One person's visualization of what can be created, just as God created man. This is the very concept or rather key to our very existence.*

*In the following pages I will attempt to address my views and outcome of being exposed to various circumstances and the hope mentioned above, but first I need to tell the story of where I came from before I attempt to address where I'm at. I am further compelled by a greater force than myself to tell of my life experiences that may help another cope or even change their quality of life for a better existence.*

*And I wish above all things you prosper and be in good health...*

*St John*

Chapter 1: 'Childhood Memories'

Growing up I could remember even at a very young age, the smell of those good old greens and neck bones cooking in that tiny two-bedroom house at least two blocks away. Of course there was also the smell of the good old crusty corn bread my mother, Helen, cooked to go with the greens and neck bones, and I could never forget the days she included the infamous lima beans. But I preferred the juicy fried chicken, which we rarely ate in comparison to the beans. You could smell the aroma before you could even see the little house on 1813 Bramble Street in second ward. As the windows and doors always remained open, it was a small close nit neighborhood with no more than about seven houses on a gravel-paved street. There were about two houses next to us, two behind us, and three across the street. On the corner sat a small neighborhood tavern that my mother referred to as a beer joint, and further down the street was Chuong Luong's grocery store.

I recall the peeling white paint making the appearance of an old grayish colored house as a chair and a few plants sat along the wooden rail framing around the front porch. One plant in particular my mother called a *mother-in-law-tongue*, sat in a tall white metal porcelain pot. It remained alive well into my adulthood. I loved to sit on the front porch, mostly when it rained but as the rain would get harder I would find myself looking out from the screen door or window singing a little song my father taught me. "Rain, rain, go away come back another day", as I could only imagine my father and his siblings growing up in Louisiana singing the same tune and enjoying the rain as I. Watching one drop fall after another, I would always end up most relaxed and ultimately asleep. But on the more sunny days I ended up outside almost daily.

In the front yard sat an old rusty swing, which I wished would last forever. As I swung back and forth on that old shaky squeaking swing looking up at the sky and trees swaying, I could feel a cool breeze on my face which was so wonderful that it made me feel like I was on top of the world. But on the side of the house was what I thought of as sheer terror.  It was our large beautiful black furry, and yet somewhat viscous dog named Rex.  My parents kept him chained and I was so terrified that I always walked all the way around to the other side, or close to the end of the chain-link fence just to avoid being close to Rex.  One day I recall being chased by Rex as I had gotten too close and if the chain had not stopped him, I knew he would have bitten me.  Just the sound of those terrifying growls wreaks sheer fear over my whole soul.  Even today I still fear most animals and I attribute this phobia to my childhood memories of our dog Rex.  In my eyes he was no doubt a ferocious animal and I will never forget the fear I felt back then.  All I could see were those huge teeth backing me into the fence.  Helen would sometimes call him away while reiterating, "Here Rex, Here boy.  I don't know why y'all so scary.  The only reason Rex bit Velma was because she was teasing him."  All I knew was he had bit my older sister, and from the looks of things he would love to bite me too.

In the backyard sat the outhouse, garden, and the clubhouse that my oldest brother Fred built.  Not long before Fred built that clubhouse, the landlord built an indoor commode or rather rest room in the house.  I remember how happy I was when the landlord put in the commode.  I recall one night while sitting in the outhouse in the dark; I saw scary shadow like images, as cockroaches scattering the yard.  I was deathly afraid of the dark and the roaches.  My mother was flabbergasted as our neighbor, Mrs. Puerez stepped on the insects with her bare feet.  It seemed pitch dark as I continually called out to my mother for assurance that I was not alone.  My vivid imagination would run wild as the outhouse hovered over me like an empty haunted house filled with ghost lurking all around me as I looked up in the dark.  It seemed as though the only visible light would shine down was from the moon and hundreds of bright stars, which lined the sky.  It seems like I have not seen that many stars since my childhood.

The only nice view in that backyard was my Daddy's garden.  We had a peach tree and a fig tree.  I loved to eat the figs right off the tree, if I could beat the birds to the sweet ripe ones.  My father further planted all kind of beans, peppers, mustard greens, and lots of okra and

tomatoes.  I loved to eat the tomatoes with a little salt.  Out of all the
food my parents cooked I loved my Dad's gumbo the best, which was
filled with okra and tomatoes of course.  Being an extremely selective
eater was not very beneficial considering our most meager situation to
say the least.

As I recall at about the tender age of five, I refused to eat
everything that had been cooked mainly those lima beans and greens.
One morning I recall Daddy fixed hot water cornbread and cooked it like
pancakes in the iron skillet.  My sister Sophia loved it as she loaded
butter and sugar on top of the small yellow pancake-like patties.  As I sat
still just merely looking at the food as Daddy said, "You better eat girl,
and you are not getting up from the table until you eat".  I just sat in
dismay as Sophia exclaimed, "Eat it, it is so good.  I put some butter and
sugar on it".  After putting as much butter and sugar as I possibly could
on the bread, I still could barely eat it.  I took a couple of bites and
Daddy looked a bit upset as I just sat there.  Finally Sophia said she
would eat it and I happily pushed it over to her.  A few days passed and I
became very ill with flu-like symptoms, and refused food altogether.
Needless to say my family was worried, as I did not eat for a few days,
and they had grave concerns that my life might be at risk.  I recall feeling
deep agonizing hunger pains from the very depths of my soul while lying
in the bed almost lifeless.  After starvation became a possible threat, my
father became desperate.  As he gave me a slice of bread and exclaimed,
"Eat the bread, Please Eat it.  If you do not eat, I am going to take you to
the hospital," he would walk off in disgust advising my mother of his
intentions as he started getting ready to catch the bus and take me to the
hospital.  My father never really hesitated to take any of us to the doctor
at the first sign of illness.  I suppose his actions were partial related to his
father's early death, which could have been avoided by possibly seeking
early medical help.  Nonetheless I still would not eat.  Then my oldest
sister, Velma, gave me a saucer of catsup.  Finally when my father was
about to pick me up and throw me over his shoulder, I started to dip the
bread into the catsup.  As my sister started to shout through the house,
"she's eating, she's eating!"  The whole family stood over me with huge

smiles all around as it was almost frightening. And to this day I love catsup and anything with tomatoes in it, is inevitably my favorite food.

I can still remember waiting and anticipating those green tomatoes in Daddy's garden to turn red. It seemed like an eternity, as I always ate them before they were completely red. I remember watching my Dad sprinkle salt on everything from tomatoes to watermelon. I no doubt picked up the habit and shook the stuff on every piece of fresh food I ate. I put salt on tomatoes of course and apples, oranges, peaches, cantaloupe, and any other sweet fruit. It became a normalcy in the way I ate my fruit.

I recall Daddy planting his garden often and I loved those times. Just being outside with the tall trees and birds humming was a beautiful feeling of comfort. Sitting and watching my father pick his fresh green beans, pinto beans, green and red peppers, okra, and the tomatoes, which always seemed to be last. I guest tomatoes took longer because they were the only good things in the garden, at least from my point of view.

On the other side of the Daddy's garden was the clubhouse that my brother Fred built. Although the clubhouse did not last as long as the garden, due to my mother ordering Fred to tear it down after my most unfortunate incident.

This incident occurred one autumn day while I was sitting outside in the clubhouse. As the leaves and twigs continued to fall from the trees, I decided to sit on the edge of the clubhouse. Within a few moments after I sat down I began to feel very uncomfortable. I started to walk toward the house, and as I got closer and closer to the house the pain became more excruciating. I cried for my mother and hence, my mother spent most of the afternoon trying to figure out what was wrong with me. Finally, shamefully pointing to my backside, my mother in total shock and dismay carefully turned me over onto her lap. After looking closely, I felt her pulling something. Then saying "Oh my God, this girl has a splinter in her but. Hilton, look at what I pulled out of this girl. Tell Fred to tear that thing down right now, right now, I just pulled a piece of splintered wood out of this girl." To this day I cannot figure out how the splinter was so precise, but needless to say it was a most extraordinary event. While the commotion was going on, my brother Fred began to hesitantly tear down the infamous clubhouse. My mother, Helen was more of the order giver of the house, I guest she was just good at conveying an opinion. While my Dad was more of the quiet-type, merely enforcing the rules when necessary.

Everyone called my mother by her first name, Helen, even her five children attempted to pronounce Helen but ended up muttering, "Halan". People who were not familiar with my family seemed bewildered and would often exclaim, "You call your mother Helen, why don't you all call your mother by her first name". Back then I could not give any response, and answered with only a shrug of the shoulders because it puzzled me as well. After I reached adulthood, I finally figured, when Fred was born and heard Helen's older sister's children calling her 'Helen' whom she help raise, he just followed suit and called her 'Helen' as well. I guess Helen just never felt the need to correct the problem as everyone referred to Helen's mother, Addie, as 'Mother'. Thus, this tradition continued, and somehow all my mother's children managed to pick up the habit all the way down to her last child, me. We all knew what Helen meant, 'Mother', just as Daddy meant Daddy. Hence we referred to my parents as Helen and Daddy.


My father eventually developed a serious heart condition before I reached school age, and was unable to continue working as a laborer. Even though the VA categorized his illness as non-service connected, he did receive a very small compensation check but was unable to support the family. Upon his diagnosis, Helen returned to the work force as a maid while I stayed home with Daddy until I became school age. My mother sometimes only made five dollars a day, and that was what one might term as poor with a long o.

After my mother returned to work, I recall the days I spend with my Dad as very serene and pleasant. I loved being with my Dad during the daytime. Once I was talking with my Dad about the tooth fairy as I started to figure out the logistics of her existence, "Daddy" I exclaimed in the mist of my deep thought. "Yea", he said. "Is the tooth fairy real". "Girl what you talking about, I'm trying to read", as he pulled and turned the page of his paper appearing to ignore my every word and move. "Well, if the tooth fairy is real, how does she know if you put a real tooth under your pillow or not. I mean I could put anything under my pillow, and so how could she tell if it's a tooth or not Daddy? I don't think she is real Daddy", as I quietly decided to put the tooth fairy to the test. Hence, I proceeded to put a button underneath my pillow while my Dad apparently looked on. I left the room and upon returning I was pleasantly surprised with some small change. I was so excited as I exclaimed, "Daddy, Daddy look I found money". Then I stopped and thought and asked, "Daddy did you put that money under my pillow"? He comely and most assuredly replied, "I don't know what you are talking about girl." " Daddy, look I found money", I announced once again. After my Dad whole heartily refused to respond to my findings. I reconsidered my thoughts on the tooth fairy being a fallacy and decided to believe in her once again. That small change was a miracle from heaven in my eyes because growing up poor definitely had its drawbacks.

During the day my Dad was very quiet, as he mostly performed chores around the house. He mainly tended to his garden, washed the clothes by hand in the wash small porcelain pan with a rub board, and then read awhile. Being poor we depended a lot on the garden as well as the chickens my father sometimes raised. But we mainly depended on the goodwill of other people to survive. We would also make a trip every once in awhile to the downtown grocery store. I remember seeing lots of tall buildings, traffic, and crowds of people. As we would make our way to Weingartens to purchase a small package of meat mainly for seasoning, but sometimes Helen would buy whole chicken fryer. I recall walking in what I thought was a huge grocery store with a department store located in the same building. A partition, which was a large sliding door, separated the two places, as sometimes we would walk through the doorway from the grocery store to the department store. I loved to look at the beautiful dolls as my heart yearned for one, but we were unable to afford to purchase anything from that store.  Eventually the department store closed down, but the grocery store remained open until my teenage years.  The floor was made of long planks of wood and one day while we were in the store I asked my parents for water.  I faintly remember a fountain that my mother put me up to and I recall not wanting to drink, as the fountain appeared rather dirty and old.  I later recalled drinking from another fountain as I was taking too long and my mother pulled me saying, "Girl that's enough now, let's go".  I remembered the water being so cold and good; I did not want to stop drinking.

As we could barely afford anything, we were blessed with varying charitable assistance through the years.  Sometimes we would receive a box of commodities which included lima beans, rice, butter, cheese, and some others items.  My father would cut the cheese into small pieces and eat it by itself like candy, while I would look through the box of commodities for something good to eat.  Commodities were some type of a charitable or government program, which provided food for low-income families.  Also, one of my mothers' nephews, Herman, would come by and help us as well.  I even remember one day Herman stopped by and brought us a sofa and a box of clothes.  Hand-me downs were a way of life in our house, as I rarely recall new clothes. Sometimes Mrs. Bell, a long time family friend who lived next door to our church would buy us a new dress for Easter.  She was like the grandmother I never knew, an older lady who loved for us to stop by after church and visit.  I recall she once bought me a beautiful chiffon yellow dress with lace, a fluffy petticoat underneath, and a sash, that I loved to wear on Sunday's.  Sometimes my Aunt Katie would make my sister and I the same dress, and on rare occasions my mother purchased us the same dress.  Helen loved to dress us alike as we were only two years apart.  Other charitable organizations like the Goodfellas delivered a box of toys on Christmas, and I always managed to get that one special doll.  It seemed like it was purchased just me.  On Christmas we would normally receive one gift each, but sometimes an extra one would be in the box of toys.

My first Christmas that I recall rather vividly was a doll, with long hair that I loved to comb. I would eventually make a little dollhouse with blankets covered over a couple of chairs. As I would crawl underneath the blanket where I would sometimes hide and make believe. I also made believe an old cigar box was a refrigerator as I played with my dolls in which I conveniently named one doll Lovera. Of course that was the brand name on the cigar box. My sister, Sophia, and I made conversation with imaginary people. We loved to play in the old light green cabinet with the pull out porcelain counter top, as well as doors on the top and bottom where our make believe characters lived. Miss Pookie Lock lived there with her family and that was where the fun began. We knocked on the cabinet doors and opened them back and forth, as we pretended our dolls were her children while asking Miss Pookie Lock to let her children come out and play. Mostly we played with Miss Pookie Lock on rainy days or days when we could not go outside and play.

During the summer as well as the weekends was when our family stayed outdoors quite a lot. As I loved to play outside in my red boots someone had given us, and was sad the day my mother gave them away as they had gotten too small. I would wake up get dressed and put on my red boots, and within a few moments I would scurry outside. Playing in the dirt with my sister was a favorite outdoors pastime when we were not playing on the rusty swing. I would find old coke bottle tops and pack them with dirt and a little water. One day my sister dared me to eat the mud pie, and as I would put it in my mouth she would yell, "Helen, Nanette is eating dirt". It was pretty horrible tasting as I would spit it out immediately. Finally, my mother forbade us from ever playing in the dirt again.

Charles, Sophia and myself were the three youngest siblings, and on rainy days when we were stuck in the house all day long sometimes trouble would follow. One day as we decided to tear up paper, and Charles whom is four years my senior was supposedly in charge of watching Sophia and I. I started to eat a piece of the paper, and Charles looked over and started yelling and crying. As my mother hurried into the room, and made me spit it out. Whenever my brother was upset, his emotional reaction would always be to pace from the front of the house to the back of the house crying. On the opposite end of the spectrum was cool and calm, Sophia, only two years older than myself preferred watching soap operas instead of playing. I would beg her to play dolls, but she would always sneak off and leave me playing alone. I would always find her sitting on the sofa watching the soap operas. But in between my pleading for her to play with me, I started to notice something very odd. I noticed all our dolls toes and some of the fingers were missing. As I often wondered about this mystery, but would not learn until we became adults, that my sister had a serious habit. We would laugh about it years later, as I learned she would bite off the tip ends of our dolls digits while watching the soaps. I would eventually wish I had kept my slightly fragmented most memorable dolls, but during our teenage years we decided to donate them to charity.

One other particular event while growing up that stands out in my mind with my sister was most hair-raising, and I mean literally a hair-raising event. As Sophia decided to hide and comb her hair in the bathroom for the first time, she would ultimately end up tangling up the comb in the bangs of her hair. She would call my name crying over and over again pleading for me to help her, and of course I had no idea what to do. She exclaimed, "Nanette, Nanette, come here and watch the bathroom door for me. Please don't tell Helen, but this comb won't come out of my hair. If she ask for me, just tell her I'm still using the rest room, but I'm coming". While my mother continued to call for Sophia while asking me what she was doing in the bathroom so long, I ran back and fourth, "She's coming, she said she coming". Finally, as I had become an accessory my mother burst through the door and was enraged with the situation, "What are you doing in here girl? What in the world have you done. I cannot believe this. How in the world could you get this comb tangled up in your hair like this"? She would try for more than an hour to untangle the comb from my sister's bangs while telling me I would receive a spanking just for covering for her. My mother said I ran back and forth lying for my sister and that was not acceptable.  Helen tried to remove the comb, but to no avail as she eventually decided to cut Sophia's bangs.  I will never forget that spanking as I felt it was not my fault, and I definitely did not deserve punishment for being merely an innocent bystander.  But I now know my mother's strong hand of discipline probably saved me from any future accessory behavior.  But discipline was seldom needed as we spent most of our time playing and in make believe land.  I recall how my brother Charles exhibited great intelligence as some of his creativity would only be preceded by my older brother, Fred.  As Helen often compared it to how Fred would make him a pulpit and preach a very creative sermon in his younger days.

Charles's creativity would cause him to engage in deep thought, as he would not have time to aggravate me or play boxing with my dolls. Our most beloved resident mad scientist would walk from the front of the house to the back crying because he could not find his socks, or some other thing misplaced during an experiment.  He loved running up behind me grabbing my hand and then rubbing my knuckles until I would scream for my mother.  "Halan, Halan, Make Charles stop", as I attempted to pull away to no avail.  Finally my mother would come over and say, "Boy leave that girl alone, go on now leave her alone I said". As he would run away sniveling, I would be in tears from the mere aggravation of trying to get away from him.

The best days were when Charles put on his plays.  He would hang a sheet in the living room as the stage curtain, and inform myself as well as Sophia of our lines.  Within minutes we proceeded with the play, and were expected to know the lines. Charles hung a piece of rope across the room with sheets draped over the rope.  He would announce,  "there will be a play at 2 o'clock in the living room theater".  I cannot recall the name of the play, but it entailed a ship in a stormy sea.  Then he would pull back the curtain and we started the play on his queue. Charles would get so mad at me as I would not be able to memorize my lines, and he had to yell out my lines to me during the performance.  He would sway the ship back and forth that he made from a combination of a large square board with a sofa pillow underneath the center, while steering with some large round object. Helen and Daddy watched and enjoyed his creative abilities, and were so proud as they loved boasting about how smart all their children were.

As Charles was always experimenting and creating, one day he decided to make some cheese. I believe he invented his own recipe from reading an old set of encyclopedias that one of his many admiring teachers gave him. He put the invention on the bottom shelve of the teal green cabinet in the kitchen to age. But Helen kept getting a whiff of the foul odor throughout the house, "Something is smelling in this house. What is that smell and where is it coming from". As Helen had us all trying to find the smell, I finally ran across the moldy concoction, "Here it is, it is this green and white stuff wrapped in this mess cloth". As she forced Charles to dispose of it, "Boy get that stuff out of here right now, and do not eat it. You will fool around and hurt your self eating that molded and spoiled food". As Charles exclaimed how the aging molded cheese would not hurt you to no avail, as Helen made him dispose of it. On another occasion, my brother decided to make me a pair of shoes with my father's old shoe equipment. Though they were made of cardboard and thumbtacks, it was a rather neat invention for a young child. He measured my feet most precisely while cutting out his pattern most carefully, and coloring them with his crayons. I was rather proud of my shoes until one day while walking they completely fell apart; he tried fixing them but would eventually give up, as the cardboard would just keep coming apart. He further spoke of how he could make milk from potatoes and nuts, but this ingenious invention would never materialize as Helen would not take a chance on another thing as she feared their might be more objectionable odors involved. Little did my mother know that I would be purchasing those same milks that my brother spoke of making at the grocery store many years later. If we had only knew his talent, maybe we could have nurtured him a little bit more to reach his full potential, rather than another "dream deferred".

Helen often said how smart her children were and thought her and my father boasted a bit too much, as she felt everyone grew weary of hearing about us. She further always spoke of the importance my father placed on our education.  His passion was for our lives to be better than what he had experienced in his life.  I feel this passion stemmed from his childhood and life experiences, he knew we would have much better opportunities with an education than without one.  Although I was very young when my father died, I was able to learn things about him from my older brother, Charles, who basically confirmed the fact that Daddy was not able to finish school.  He said our grandfather, Cecil, made my father and his brothers work in the fields cutting and caning sugar.  My father had to quit school at a very young age, as he only made it to third grade.  Charles further advised me of a story Daddy shared about my grandfather's untimely death.  As my father spoke to Charles very slowly and rather somberly stating, "When I was about fifteen, my father, Cecil had been very ill for a few days.  Finally, he was getting worse and I hopped on my horse, and rode and rode as fast as I could to get to town.  By the time I returned with the doctor, it was too late and the doctor said my father died from a ruptured appendix.  He said if we had came a little sooner, maybe he could have saved Cecil."  Although my father rarely talked about himself, I do remember asking my father about why he was so poor and he replied, "After my father died, people just came in and walked away with our furniture and other things of value."  I tried to envision the facts surrounding Cecil's untimely departure, and what happened to their valuables.  I eventually came to a conclusion that Cecil probably owed a lot of people in his business circle, as his compensation for sugar cane was probably not very fair.  As they were just struggling to survive, as well as a possibility of overzealous indulgence or an occasional cocktail to just remain grounded in the important things such as family.

My father indulged in an occasional drink like most of his siblings, but he would only drink in the late evening hour.  I recall whenever there would be a death in my father's family, all the men would sit around quietly as they passed around the bourbon.  I personally did not know much about my Dad but I did know I loved him dearly and he most certainly loved me.  As my father would eventually pass away when I was only ten years old.

A few years before my father passed away my eldest brother, Fred, would volunteer for the Marines.  Prior to leaving at the tender age of seventeen, my brother worked at Kim's grocery store.  The owners and his family loved my brother dearly.  Some nights after arriving home from work, he would take us outside directly in front of the house onto the shell-paved street.  He played the magician standing directly underneath the corner street light while pulling kool-aid and candy from behind his back, as the crickets sang and the fireflies circled around the street light.  We called the candy 'the good stuff', and my big sister Velma always hid it in a small paper bag underneath her bed or pillow eating it as she pleased, and hiding it from us as we only received a couple of small pieces.  As I found the stash of candy under her bed one day she would exclaim, "Where did you find this candy and what are you doing in my room?  And stay out of my things."  As I stood and kept badgering her until she finally broke, and gave up one measly piece a candy.

Fred left for the marines right after his eighteenth birthday when I was only four years old, but I can remember when he received the uniform.  He would look in the mirror and adjust his hat, as Fred appeared very handsome and proud of the fact he would fight for his country.  Helen and Daddy gave Fred a going away party; all his friends and some of the family came.  His friends were really nice to me, and one of the girls who liked my brother carried me around for most of the party.  Finally after she got tired and put me down, I cried and cried and Helen's sister, Aunt Katie asked,  "What's wrong with you honey".  I did not respond but Helen knew what the problem was as she just sat me on her lap, and I was quiet the rest of the evening.  Being the youngest and sometimes referred to as the cutest as two of siblings were at least ten or more years older, one could expect to be a little spoiled.

As I sensed my parents made a significant change after Fred left for the marines.  Although we prayed before he left, Helen appeared to stay on her knees praying much more often and for longer periods of time. I further found my father often praying on bended knees morning and night as well as reading his bible. Once my parents were writing letters to Fred, I would eventually write him one on my own. While sitting on the porch one breezy day as the trees swayed slowly from side to side, I started looking at the clouds in the sky. It was as though I was having an angelic experience and a soft melody dropped from the heavens. "Lord please bring Fred back home someday", and I sang that same verse a couple of times while the chorus included a downward scale of singing "someday" over and over. It was my prayer to God as I felt much comfort from missing my older brother so very much. As the breeze felt like God was breathing a sigh of peace within the very debts of my soul, I had never felt such peace. Afterwards I would never worry about Fred again as I knew he would return home safe. It was no doubt a wonderful experience and what I thought was a lovely song, but it was hard to convince everyone else to bass in the glory I felt. First I told everyone I had wrote a song for Fred, then I proceeded to ask Velma, my older sister, to write it on paper. I wanted it to be written on music paper and with musical notes, but I did not know what anything was called. Thelma had transferred to San Jacinto High School, and had started taking music lessons. As parents had recently purchased a violin for my sister, and my brother would send home a little money. He thought maybe he could help my sister one day pay for college. So I had been watching her read the sheet music, while practicing on her violin. After about thirty minutes of a four-year-old trying to describe a musical note, Velma finally clicked as she most kindly drew notes and wrote the words I shyly sang.

Years later I would reminisce about the pass, and wondered if my brother even remembered receiving the letter. I did finally have a chance to ask him, as he did not recall the actual letter. But he did respond, "That's why I made it back, while so many of the other guys who left with me didn't." I advised him that not only was I praying, but also his leaving literally changed Helen and Daddy. I recalled how Helen and Daddy would wake up in the wee hours of the morning and night for prayer. My father would always get on his knees at night and get up early in the morning as he usually did, but it seemed like something started to change after my brother enlisted in the Marines.

About a year before my father passed, Helen received a better
paying housekeeping job at the YMCA, we were able to fix somewhat
better meals.  Daddy would fix breakfast for everyone and after fixing
breakfast he would sit in the chair next to the small table in the kitchen.
As I would watch him put on his glasses he bought from the corner drug
store, and then read his small catholic bible cover to cover every single
morning.  I later revealed to my brother how his leaving affected our
parents, and Fred was not surprised, as revealed to me how upon his
return from the Marines Helen would go out at night looking for him.
Fred was in his mid-twenties as Helen would walk up to the
neighborhood nightclub, and ask him to come out.  I was not surprised
either as she did whatever she could to steer all of her children in the
right direction.  As Helen often exclaimed,  "I would die to save any one
of my children."
     I know my parents loved all their children more than life itself,
but they lived in a time where fighting spouses was very much more
acceptable.  I recall Helen had gone out visiting friends one evening, and
left us with my father.  She later returned to find my sister and I hiding
under a blanket behind a chair.  Daddy had been drinking and was
growling like a monster, and laughed as we ran and hid while screaming
in sheer fright.  Finally, we thought we had a sign of relief as Helen
returned, and not a moment to soon for my sister Sophia and myself.  We
hurriedly ran to her clinging to her dress tail until the shouting began.
"Hilton, why are you teasing those children like that", my mother
shouted.  Daddy said,  "Ah, I am not scaring them and move back."  "I
said stop it Hilton, and leave them alone", Helen stated again.  Then the
pushing and shoving started, and before you knew it my parents were in
a heated fight.  Although Helen and Daddy sounded and looked as if they
were having knock out drag out fights, I never saw any bruises or visible
marks on either one of them.  Even though they rarely fought, I still

wondered why and tried to rationalize some years later. After much evaluation of their complexities on the inside and outside, I know my parents were extremely intelligent but inside were two victims of the time. My mother always spoke of her straight A's at Phyllis Wheatley High School. Daddy only went to third grade as he was forced to cane sugar in the swamps of Louisiana for his family's survival. But he somehow managed to teach himself how to read and write, and even attended Texas Southern University for Shoe Making and Repair. How extraordinary that two most intelligent people would appear to exhibit to me such frustration.

They were frustrated as the lack of opportunities for Blacks, lack of opportunities for themselves, and my parents could only hope and pray that their children would end up in much better circumstances than being frustrated and poor. My parents were merely doing the best that they could to raise up successful adults. Sometimes my parents were rather strict, but I later realized they were only trying to protect us. They were trying to keep us from drugs, alcohol, and all the other evils that would prevent us from being the best we could be. Throughout all the hard times, we were our parents' whole life and they spent a large amount of time raising and molding us into productive human beings. I truly believe if my father had an opportunity to attend school, he would have been in very different circumstances. I believe my father just as my mother wanted and dreamed of doing great things. I felt I was a mirror image of my father as I later developed the same quest he had. The quest for knowledge that he had been deprived, by not being able to obtain an adequate education. I further felt this was one of the reasons my father drank. As I recall my father reading his Bible and praying, I can't help but believe he lacked all hope for himself. He had no hope for his future existence, but somehow he did live and instill hope for us. I believe if my father had hope for his future, he would have been delivered from his alcoholism. I was eventually delivered from alcoholism, through the gospel of Jesus Christ by confessing my sins, and asking God to give me strength. It further was from my mothers' continued prayers that I was delivered. Sometimes I wonder if my father actually knew the great healing power that God instilled in his very soul.  But still my father was a great inspiring force in my life.  When I experienced any painful incidents in my life, I would always remind myself of my father's expectations for his children's life.  Whenever I would feel less than adequate or felt like giving up, I thought of my father.  I knew he would want the best for me, to be proud of me, and I knew I could be that great person my father wanted me to be.  As I knew my parents loved us deeply and we all loved them as well.

The memory that seems most prevalent in my mind about Daddy was our long walks as I later came to cherish that time we spent together.  While walking he liked to sing a tune to me, "Doe, Doe, Tee, Babe".  That's about the only part of the song I remember, but I do recall some very distinct French he spoke such as, "Parlez vous Francais?"  I would respond by saying, "What does that mean Daddy"?  "Do you speak French" as he smiled and called me nutty pony, and he would continue, "Can you say thank you, Merci Boeuque".  He spoke French so distinctly as I found it was the language they spoke in France, after taking a year of the French language in high school.

I vividly remember our long walks to the neighborhood store.  We sometimes took the scenic or long routes, as I thought my Dad loved to walk.  But later found there was a reason why my Dad walked rather slowly and looking downward.  Years later after my son was born he asked me, "Why do you walk with your head always hung down?"  As I thought a moment I finally realized, it stemmed from my childhood walks with my Dad many years ago.  My Dad always looked down at the ground as we were walking, and I recalled asking my Dad a similar question, "What are looking for Daddy"?  He advised, "I found some money one day when I was walking so I always look to see if I can find some more".  So needless to say I started looking down from that day on, just like my Dad.  We rarely talked but walked quietly with our heads looking downward, and sometimes pushed the dirt over with our feet so we would not miss any small coins.

While my Dad was a rather quiet man, my mother, Helen was a bit more outgoing.  As she appeared to be rather stubborn, and spoke her opinion on most issues and often times would not listen to any other reasoning. Helen refused to let Daddy have the last word and visa versa. I often felt most of my parents disputes could have been avoided, if Helen would have just let Daddy win. I guest I felt that way because Helen was sober, and Daddy did not start arguments unless he had a drink or two. The only time Daddy talked or acted different was when he sometimes had a drink at night. He would always buy a pint of Jack Daniel's or other similar name brands of alcohol in the afternoon. He kept his pint bottle of alcohol in the closet of his bedroom, and did not touch it until the sun went down.

Sometimes I felt he would have given up the urge to fight if Helen had just keep quiet, but my mother did not take any flack from anyone. Basically none of her children challenged her as she commanded respect, Helen always said she would never let anyone run over her including her children. As my parents continued their disagreements, they never really realized how it might have been affecting their children.

Sometimes they even quarreled a bit when my oldest brother Fred was small, as Helen told us a story of someone trying to rescue her from my father. My mother had decided my father was staying out a little too late at the corner tavern where my father sometimes stopped after work. She approached him and asked him to come home now, as they were walking down the street arguing, a neighbor, Mr. Mike asked, "Hey what's going on, do you need some help Helen?" Helen simply responded by saying, "If we want to fight you leave us alone, he's my husband so stay out of it". Apparently Helen felt it was something between her and my father. My brother Fred's general rule was to never interfere with a husband and wife having a dispute because they might turn on you.

But through it all, my Dad was a loving father. As I recall the days just after I had my traumatic experience of kidney infection, Daddy insisted on giving me medicine even if I just merely attempted to close my eyes to take a nap. While I can't recall very much about that night I was rushed to the hospital with the infection, I was told how I was afraid of everyone. I did not recognize anyone as I was delirious and was told I screamed and tried to run as my brother, Fred, attempted to hand me an orange, " Stay away from me, help, someone help me", I cried while burning up with fever. My parents immediately rushed me to the emergency room as I eventually recalled the long and hazy ride to the ER, a shot on my backside, and the horrible tasting medicine I had to take until my next visit to the doctor. Although the doctor tested and released me from his care the next few weeks, my Daddy still kept medicine in the house he bought at the drug store especially for me. The medicine tasted horrible and was called "Baby Percy". Whenever I came home and just sat too long my father would exclaim, "Get the Baby Percy, she's about to go to sleep." After awhile I tried to force myself not to nap after school just so Daddy would not make me take that horrible tasting medicine. Helen would sometime help me out by saying, "Hilton leave that girl alone. She's just tired and sleepy from her long day at school."

Daddy certainly had his days of overly nurturing me as I guess I had my days of smothering him as well. I recall one warm Midsummer Day, I decided to teach my father proper penmanship. Daddy had to quit school in the third grade, so his writing was not as good as it could have been. Although I doubt my penmanship was anywhere near proper I still exclaimed, "Daddy, I'm going to teach how to write in cursive. First, let us start with the letter A. Now write it just like I did. Very good, now write a B". By the time I reached the letter C, Daddy had gotten frustrated with me and looked over the top of his newspaper and said, "Girl go on, I'm trying to read". After about two or three times of telling me, he finally yelled, and his yell was enough to scare me into obedience. As I look back on that event, I guess I might have made my Dad feel bad.

Although my father never really spanked me, his yell made up for it. His voice was very deep and strong, and it carried a force that could not be reckoned with. His voice could always put fear deep down within my very soul that made me tremble like a leaf. As my mother always said I was just a timid child, I would later figure out why.

Although it was not very often, I truly hate admitting how my father sometimes frightened me when he drank, as I would quench. Otherwise, I just loved to be with him even more than being with my mother. Every time my father raised his voice I ran away shaking, and put my two fists underneath my chin and hid until I felt it was safe again. One day I became so engulfed with fear until, I imagined my whole family were monsters disguised as humans.

I often feel this was the first onset of many dark and unhappy events in my life. I remember watching everyone for days as if I were watching a movie. I sat as everyone moved back and fourth in the kitchen. It was like a dream, a bad dream I could not awaken from. Then, finally, my sister Velma asked, "What's wrong Nanette, why are you so quiet and just sitting there watching us like that? Come on, what's wrong?" After a few moments of hesitation, I finally responded, "well I thought, you were all monsters". Velma let out a big laugh while Helen responded, "Now why would think such a thing. Look, we are not monsters. We are just like you". Needless to say I did get over that fear, but there would be many more incidents to overcome.

The fear of my own family was one with very mixed and mostly unsubstantial emotions. I loved my family very much, but little insignificant events became gradually heightened after the onset of a most unfortunate incident that occurred during my first year of elementary school. This incident was not one that would correct itself so easily, and would be the main source and cause of some most devastating events during my teenage as well as young adult life.

The elementary school Helen wanted us to attend was in third ward. My mother started all her children in first grade; none of us went to kindergarten. During my first year of school, we had to ride the city bus because we lived in second ward. I remember that first day very, very well, because my brother, Charles who was the oldest managed to somehow get us quite lost. Even though we were about a couple of blocks from the school, Charles walked my sister Sophia, and myself back and forth down the same street. He would walk two blocks, then turnaround saying no it's the other way and turn again. Finally, after about ten times of walking in a circle, Sophia decided not to turnaround anymore and we finally arrived at school. We would make it to school about two hours late, tired, and dripping with sweat. Also I recall feeling very nervous that first day, and I remember how huge the small hallways appeared to be that day.

Helen had made arrangements with my first grade teacher, Mrs. Admons, to stay with me after school as Charles and Sophia did not get out until later. Since they were a couple of grades higher than I, their dismissal was about two hours later. Often times Mrs. Admons left the classroom, and I would sit there alone until Charles came to get me. I never really noticed she left early until one day while sitting in my classroom, a young boy came into the room. He appeared to be a few years older than I and proceeded to ask strange and personal questions and before I knew it, his hand made its way under my dress. At that time, I did not know words like molestation or child abuse even existed. And although I attempted to block this event out of my mind, it was and is an unforgettable event that still haunts my very existence. I have come to the reality that I was in fact molested at the tender age of six. This boy was not just a boy but in fact a monster, far worst than the monsters I envisioned my family to be. Immediately after I told my mother what had happened, she examined me and was furious. Not long afterwards my parents demanded a meeting with the principal, Mrs. Admons, and the other little girl whom the boy was chasing when he stopped and noticed me. We went from classroom to classroom trying to find the boy. I thought we found him, but the sixth grader adamantly denied the incident even occurred, and I knew who he was and what he had done. But after all his denying, arguing, and crying, I was so confused and afraid that I stopped talking. Deep down inside I guess I was terrified at the thought he would come back and get me if they punished him, just like he told me he would. I further recalled how he pulled out a knife while he threatened me. I do not really know if he ever touched the other little girl, as she ran around laughing when he chased her. I do feel I was an easy defenseless target, as I was sitting quietly when he approached me.

After the meeting Helen advised me to leave and go to another classroom or the office, if my teacher ever left me alone again. Although I deliberately put this event out of the forefront of my mind for many years, I feel it was never subconsciously forgotten and made me into a very timid and fearful child. I feared people I did not know and sometimes people I knew very well. It further created a lot of confusion in my adult life as I made very bad decisions in my relationships. I feel this event was no doubt the primary cause of the bad choices I made in choosing friends, which would result in many failed relationships. I often think how this may have contributed in a large way to some of my feelings of insecurities. But over time I continued to develop a great fear in my heart of all people, mainly men that catapulted into feelings of adult insecurity. As I would remain rather shy and quiet, and I very rarely talked.

Almost immediately following the molestation incident, the teacher continued to leave me scared out of my wits in the classroom alone. Helen quickly decided it was time to move. She moved to third ward, so she would not be far from the school. I guest she felt more comfortable as she or my father would be able to pick us up from school. Although it was a good idea, it still was not a safeguard against the cycle of abuse.

The first house we moved to was on York Street, but we moved within a few weeks, as Helen did not like the area. I did recall running around and playing and jumping up and down in a bunk bed of one the neighbors' houses on York Street. Afterwards Helen was furious, and told us never to go inside stranger's homes. Helen had become overly protective of her last three children and rightfully so considering the recent abuse incident.

So we would move to yet another house nearby. The second move was even worst as we lived on Samson Street right across from a nightclub. Helen said it was a club with all kinds of goings on inside. We loved this house, as it was the largest house we had ever lived in, and my elementary school was barely a block down the street. One day my teacher Ms. Admons learned we had moved and decided to walk me home. Helen was surprised as they cordially greeted each other, even though Helen felt she was mainly responsible for molestation incident. She said Mrs. Admons should have never left me alone in the room.

"Hi, I decided to walk her home after I learned you'll had moved just down the street. How you'll doing today on this beautiful sunny afternoon", Mrs. Admons exclaimed. " Helen replied, "Oh fine, but as you can see, it is too much activity across the street with that club for these small children, and we are about to move again. But thanks for walking her home." As she walked away I recall Helen saying, "Look at her. She knew if she was not going to be in that room, she could have at least taken Nanette to the front office". Ms. Admons continued to try to make amends as I would be selected to renounce the Pledge of Allegiance at our First grade assembly to being pulled from my seat by Ms. Admons to dance to Aretha Franklin's hit song Chain of Fools at our year end party.

When we did finally move from the Samson Street house we left our antique phonograph that Helen referred to as a 'Vicktroller', and lots of my father's old records. After few years passed Helen realized they probably were collector items as they were the early 1900's items. Right next door to our house on Samson Street was a beauty shop, called Tootsie's. Tootsie and her mother worked in the shop together. First her mother would pull a hot iron comb through our hair, afterwards Tootsie pulled the hair straight with what Helen called a marcel iron. I guess this marcel iron that looked similar to a curling iron was used to attain a longer lasting silkier look. Helen enjoyed going with us and talking with the ladies, but we would move yet again to Palmer Street a few streets over. It appeared to be a much quieter neighborhood. There were a couple of middle-aged people across the street as one the lady's hand was drawn up and rather twisted as well as her leg was crippled. I often wondered what was wrong with her. Everyone called this lady, Ms. Red, as she was a rather fair-skinned lady with reddish hair. Her husband, Mr. Charlie, had to assist her in just about every move. Looking back I now know it was from a stroke as my mother's hand ended up in the same position after her massive stroke.

Another couple that lived next door to us, in a corner house would quarrel almost every night. We heard them, as they would rumble from the back of the house onto the front porch. I recall Helen and Daddy getting along well as they listened to the commotion. I guess they realized how arguing and disputes truly sounded. We eventually moved into their corner house, after the lady finally moved after a serious fight and she had to be hospitalized. Their fights were rather violent, as we feared one of them would be seriously hurt. After their last fight we recalled seeing puddles of blood on the porch from the husband stabbing her, as she returned all bandaged up and bade us goodbye after packing only a few items. We would eventually move into the house and came across various items such as dishes, clothes, and furniture left behind, as I suppose she just desperately wanted out.

On the other side of us was our neighbor, Mr. John. He was a very active man who's wife previously passed and he kept himself occupied by frequently traveling, while requesting us to keep an eye on the only huge beautiful house in the neighbor. He always dressed in his short brimmed hat with freshly shined shoes, and a Sunday suit as he had several. His house further had a huge fireplace and you could tell from the fine furnishings that he was very well off. He kept a beautifully landscaped yard with nicely trimmed hedges and beautiful flowers, and would yell to the top of his lungs if anyone even came close to walking on his lawn. "Y'all chil'ren get out of my yard now", as he always talked very fast and became enraged whenever the neighborhood kids would walk across his yard as some of the kids did it just to hear him yell. After all the yelling, one could hardly believe he was really a very nice mild mannered gentleman who mostly laughed during the entire conversation with my Mom and Dad. As he loved to sit on the large front porch encircled by banisters with his feet propped up, while listening to the baseball game almost every Sunday evening after church. He took trips to Louisiana often and would always bring us back souvenirs and gingerbread pastries that we called stage planks, and if we ever needed anything including money, we could always ask Mr. John as his response would always be don't worry about it. My mother always tried to pay him back, but sometimes he would not take it back responding, "Keep it don't worry about it". My mother would plead with him to take his money, "Oh Mr. John, no, I can't keep it". But sometimes he would insist. Years later after we moved from the neighborhood, we heard that our beloved neighbor was hit over the head and robbed while he waited for the bus. He died from the fatal blow as we later learned one of the long time incarcerated neighborhood drug addicts was released only a few days before the murder occurred.

Once we moved to the corner house on Palmer Street, my mother would start back straightening our thick fluffy hair with the hot comb herself. She started to worry about my sister and I walking around the neighborhood alone. The neighborhood had started to deteriorate, as well as the nearby fire station closed down. Passing cars would always honk, or guys would yell out of their cars at my sister and I. As it had become the norm, Helen would always tell us, "When that happens, don't even look at those guys. Just keep walking, don't pay them any attention and run as fast as you can if they come after you. And do not get in the car with them." As my mother stressed the last statement while putting the fear of God in us, we feared her repercussions more than the guys.

Helen always pressed our hair with a hot comb, and did a pretty good job considering my protestations. I hated it, as I would always squirm and dodge the hot iron as my mother moved toward the back or edge of my hairline. That comb was hot and I guess I would have preferred our beautician, Tootsie to do my hair because I did not give her any problems. I sat still, barely moving and would have been embarrassed for anyone to know how afraid I really was. Our hair was thick, long, and fluffy, and my sister, Sophia and I hated to get our hair pressed. My father's hair texture was straighter than all of his children, as I guess our hair was a more dominant frizzy hair type, but basically an intermediary combination of both our parents.

My parents tried to raise us the right way by taking us to church every Sunday, and not allowing us to go anywhere without them. But I guest they could not be with us all the time, and tragic events still continued to occur. I tried to forget most of these tragic episodes in my life but they would inevitably follow me.

Unlike first grade I made it through second as well as third grade without any major tragic incidents. In third grade I had my first Caucasian teacher, I guess it was about 1969 when integration was beginning in Houston. Almost all the Black teachers were transferred away, and only a few seemed to be left. Our elementary school included kindergarten through the fourth grade. The fifth and sixth was a few miles away on the east side, and although it was mostly Hispanic there were a few other races that resided in the area.

When I first started the third grade, the teacher put me into group one but I was later moved to group two for reading. Group two was for the in between readers, and it was very devastating to me. I suppose mainly because my best friend, Wendy, was in the first group of readers. I was so devastated that I stopped talking to Ms. Burrows. She finally would ask me what was wrong, and after voicing my opinion and following her advise of hard work and studying I finally was moved back to group one.

Wendy and I had become best friends, as we would talk almost every day after school on the phone. We talked about our very similar situations. Both of our fathers were in the VA hospitals often with heart problems. Although her father passed away first, my father followed not long afterwards. She told me they had received a lot of gifts after her father died, and they appeared to be handling the lost well.

We always stopped by the park during my father's frequent stays in the hospital. I would beg to swing real high, but as Charles pushed I would cry for my mother to make him stop. After our brief moments of escape, I recall wishing maybe the same thing would happen to my father. I thought maybe our life would be better, as Helen had told us my father felt we would do better without him. Feelings of guilt and sadness consumed me after my father passed, as I felt I caused his death just by merely thinking those thoughts. I sorely missed my father, but as I got older I came to the realization that it was not my wish. For my dear father developed serious heart problems not only from worrying about providing for his family, but also due to some noted nutritional inconsistencies. Hence, my father suffered his fatal heart attack about two years after Fred returned home from the Marines in March of 1971.

I still remember the day very vividly when Fred returned home from his voluntary enlistment service in the Marines. Helen and Daddy ran to the door elated as they and all of us hugged my brother while sobbing in shear joy. It was not anything short of a miracle that he made it back from Vietnam. After a few days I asked, "When's Fred leaving Helen". My mother happily replied, "Your brother is not leaving girl, your brother is home for good." I knew he never stayed home very long since leaving in 1964. He always re-enlisted so I was quite happy when I found he was not leaving anymore. "Oh he lives here now", I said surprisingly. "Yes, honey your brother lives here" as my mother smiled. Although I was still young when Fred returned from Vietnam, he never spoke about his experiences even after I became an adult. As I believed he preferred to try to forget the experience. We did watch the pictures he took and put on the slide projector, which included scenes from his tent barracks in what he called a foxhole to operating the flame-thrower. Although we sat with much interest and curiosity, we just merely cherished the fact he had returned safely to us.

I recall one day during his short stay with us before he wed his first wife, he made my sister, Sophia, and I Saturday morning breakfast. He further included two tall glasses of milk and neither of us liked milk very much. As I could force myself to drink it, but Sophia simply hated it. I began to drink very slowly as Fred advised very firmly, "You both have to drink that whole glass of milk and you cannot get up from the table until you do." Sophia decided very adamantly that she was not going to drink it as I timidly completed my glass while Sophia looked over and said, "I do not drink milk and I am not going to drink it." As my brother's bark was worst than his bite, she eventually escaped punishment and was allowed to leave the table free from drinking the milk. I don't recall Fred ever doing breakfast with us that included tall glasses of milk again. The next difference of opinion I recall with my oldest brother was when I opened a can of tomato sauce for my mother.

As she asked me to throw away the can, I decided to clean the sides with my fingers. I loved anything with tomatoes, and as I walked around licking the can and my fingers Fred shouted, "Somebody take that can away from her." At the time I did not understand why my brother shouted for me to stop scraping the metal can, as he probably was afraid I would accidentally cut myself on the can. But further and more importantly we were not even aware of the dangers of metal toxins. I now recall seeing the small metal particles after they fell into the can as we used the hand held opener. As my mother mostly cooked fresh vegetables, but when we did start to eat canned vegetables I do recall pouring off the excess juice except on the canned liquids. This was no doubt the kind of ill-informed eating patterns that help lead to my eventual appendectomy, not to mention the fact that I ate very little of anything healthy and I rarely drank any water.

Also, a couple of years before my father passed, my oldest sister Velma would marry, have a daughter, and start working. She was able to acquire her nurse aid certificate and was able to purchase us all Christmas gifts. My Dad received house shoes as we woke him up early that Christmas morning. He was not very pleased by us kids waking him up. Helen received a house dress or duster as they are called, Charles received a tape recorder, and Sophia a radio. I received a 8 track tape player with a tape. This would be the first Christmas, we did not receive toys from charity. We were so happy, as I recalled later that day we all recorded and sang from an old hymn book, we sang just about all the Christmas songs in the book. That night we sang from 'God Rest Ye Merry Gentleman' to Velma's solo of 'Silent Night'. Charles also made a his own rendition of 'Swing Low Sweet Chariot' that I still remember and cherish to this day. One night after all our glorious hymn recordings, Velma decided to paint her nails, the color was called 'wicked white', how ironic. I was shocked and before I realized it, I told her she was evil and wicked just like the polish. Well needless to say, I got another back hand slap, because I would not leave her alone. Sometimes my badgering worked and other times like this time, it was futile.

⚘ ⚘ ⚘ ✦ ✦ ⚘ ⚘ ⚘ ✦ ✦ ⚘ ⚘ ⚘

It would now be almost seven years since the onset of my father's heart condition, as we appeared to make more trips to the VA hospital. It seemed like we spent a lot of time at the VA hospital fishpond, on the grass having picnics, and taking pictures. But my father still refused the needed surgery for the blocked artery, and would only live another two years after my brother returned from the Marines. My mother and father prayed often and continually concerned themselves with all their children's well being and in between the unavoidable nutritional inconsistencies or bad diet due to some unknown misconceptions, my father's heart could not take anymore and just gave out. Earlier that morning after my father went to the doctor, my mother said Dr. Sarine told my father, "Well you know your going to die Mr. Broussard". Helen was so hurt and upset as she responded, "We all are going to die one day doctor, why would you say that to someone". She further told us how she recalled the doctor giving my father some black pills, which she believed triggered the fatal heart attack.

That afternoon, Fred had parked his sky blue sedan in front of our house. A truck line was directly across from our house and as he backed up he hit my brother's car. Helen ran outside yelling as she felt he could have asked my brother to move his car. My father grabbed my mother by the arm saying, "Wait a minute Helen, wait". I think he was feeling the attack coming on at that moment, and he knew it would probably be the last. As Helen walked toward the front yard and started talking to the truck driver, Daddy grabbed his chest and before he could make it to the door he fell, as Fred's wife, Bertha caught him underneath both arms. She yelled, "Somebody help, help, it's Hilton". I just stood there in shock unable to move and get help. I watched as his eyes rolled to the back of his head as Helen realized what was happening and yelled, "Oh my Lord, someone go get the ambulance". Once the ambulance drivers arrived, as they were less than a block away, they carried him to the bed where they tried to revive him by pushing on his chest. Then I watched from afar as they carried my poor father away to the ambulance, as he was probably already deceased.  Within a few minutes, I recall the phone ringing and Fred's wife answering.  I don't remember much about the call as she concealed the bad news very well. Finally, after what appeared to be an eternity Helen and Fred walked in with horrible looks on their faces, and I knew Daddy was gone.  I was so horrified and began to yell,  "No, No", and started to back up into a corner while crying quite profusely.  I was ten years old, almost eleven and to loose your parent at such a tender age or for that matter any age was certainly most devastating.  I would eventually learn that lives are cut far too short, and knew if possible I must do something to bridge the gap.  To endeavor to be that bridge in an effort to help cease most untimely deaths, because I wished no other to experience such pain far too early in their life. I had never before experienced such pain when my father passed, and could only hope I would never experience it again.

The funeral was so sad as Helen had to be pulled away from the casket with all of us crying behind her.  I was almost eleven, but what I remembered and missed most about my father was how safe I felt when he was with us.

That same school year before my father passed away I had to start fifth grade a little late, due to what I call, 'running fan on the loose'. It was one warm summer day right before school started in September of 1970 right after returning home from visiting my father, my mother and I were changing clothes in her room.  The fan was in her room and it was considered the cooler part of the house.  While passing by the fan I pulled the cord, it dropped behind me and as my mother picked it up she noticed blood. "Oh my God, this girl is bleeding", my mother exclaimed. As we immediately rushed to the emergency room via cab, I did not even feel any thing until the doctor started to stitch the heel.  I cried in excruciating pain as he did not deaden the area enough, but after awhile another doctor came in and gave me another shot.  As the doctor slowly sewed the top area of my heal he would state, "You are lucky as it just barely missed the tendon.  If it had severed the tendon you would have had much bigger troubles."

Finally, after I received my crutches, I was able to start school. My teacher advised my parents all was well, but as I arrived things appeared very different.  Students were not very nice, as it was the first year of our school system's formal racial integration I would observe the beginnings remnants of most unkind behavior, not only from the students but teachers as well.

My fifth grade teacher, Ms.Swane often talked of the Black Panthers and the KKK.  Finally, I mentioned it to my mother and father. I advised my parents how she would write out the names of these groups on the chalkboard while further elaborating with drawing and diagrams, as she resounded almost daily that the KKK let Black people join its organization and the Black Panthers do not let White people join their group.  Although I now know her teaching methods were most inappropriate, sometimes I wonder if she really thought this was appropriate teaching for fifth grade especially when we had so many other more important subjects to learn about other than promotion of specific confrontational groups. Helen and Daddy eventually came by the school to visit with her a few times and although I do not know what was said, she would eventually stop talking about the KKK and Black Panthers.  My parents felt that these were hate groups and opinions on the groups did not have any relevance in our regular educational system.

This teacher's rambling about these groups was the least of my worries, the unruly students was the main problem. After my parents came by, some of the more unseasoned students would talk about how old my parents looked.  This talk and teasing would have a most negative affect on me as a young child, I asked my mother not to come by the school anymore. My mother would never know why I would make that request as she just felt I was embarrassed of her and my father.

The students would not obey this teacher, as they exhibited very little respect for her for varied reasons including her continued push for the so called good will of the Klan.  Principal Jonston even tried talking to our class and lectured on obedience a few times, but to no avail.  I guess the students were advising their parents as well of the lesson plan, as they choose to continue to disrespect her.  We eventually started to exchange classes for a couple of our subjects in an effort by the school to regain some control as well as attain our most needed education. Our math teacher was a stern Black lady that carried a small paddle. Ms. Davis would spank based on how many questions we missed in class. One swat per wrong answer, and thank goodness I only received one. But the one I did receive hurt my feelings more than my backside. She also spanked for talking as well. Needless to say most of the students learned very fast in her classroom. Although I displayed mixed feelings about this class, I felt much more secure going to this teacher's class. As it was much quieter than Ms. Swane unruly classroom. While we mostly sat at our desk and worked on our own in Ms. Swane's class, it was no doubt a most difficult task considering all the disruptions and noise.

During the time frame of my father's death, I had missed a lot of school days. I fell behind and Ms. Swane advised I would repeat the grade. After that revelation I worked extremely hard to catch up on my studies, and needless to say I passed the fifth grade but not without experiencing yet another abuse situation. But this time it would be by the hands of my own fellow classmates.

As there was only a couple of what I term 'actual bullies', the others were merely frightened adherents to the bullies demands of the fifth grade class. They worked together to frighten students into submission, while starting fights with students who would not succumb. Kalie, the most unscrupulous class bully was a few years older than the rest of us and no doubt had experienced some type of abuse herself in more ways than one. I recall in the beginning of the semester, Kalie was rather quiet but not long after a field trip we took to the symphony, most of my turmoil started. I recall sitting speechless in the auditorium as I noticed some older children above us, possibly middle or high school, yelling down at us. Saying rude statements and the one thing I recall vividly is, "Why don't you go back to Africa". Some of our class tried yelling back, and as I did not know what to think at the time since I had never been exposed to bigotry before. But later I recall thinking why do they hate me, when they do not even know me. It was as though I was in a bad dream and could not simply awaken from. When we exited the auditorium I felt much relief, but this incident would silently haunt my subconscious as the other seemingly insignificant yet most unyielding tragic childhood events. For they stay with us for the rest of our lives in our subconscious memories. All these childhood memories that would help mold and ultimately create, and finally manifest itself into adulthood lives through our insecurities and self-hate.

&&&&&&&&&&

During class and even after school I would always try keeping to myself, but due to the fact I would not submit I became Kalie's ideal target. I even recall how she frightened us by telling us a ghost story of how she called one of her deceased relatives back from the dead. As she made the story sound so real as she spoke rather slowly, "I went into a dark room and started to call out the person's name over and over, and as I called out their name I turned around in a circle. And finally I saw the shadow of the ghost come into the room, and I started crying as I was so scared and finally I saw her and she said don't be afraid. I was just keep crying and I could not stop crying and at first I did not believe this could really happen but I saw hear." Afterwards I went home and after a couple of try's and nothing occurred, I told my mother about the story and she advised to stop believing everything you her. But Kalie was quite able to capture and frighten most of her entourage. One of their smaller group members, Hanna, would always try to start fights until I finally grew weary and challenged her while alone in the restroom. As she promised to never bother me again and started to cry, I then felt bad about the situation. I felt as though I was no better than Kalie, but I had been pushed to my limit. She would eventually run crying to Kalie, the bully of the classroom. Needless to say she was furious at my challenging one of her loyal followers as well as her authority, and one day not long afterwards payback would rear its ugly head.

One day I asked the teacher to stay behind in the classroom during recess to work on some past assignments. I was still trying to play catch-up from so much missed school after Daddy's death, so I had to work extra hard to assure I would be promoted. But to my surprise Kalie decided to stay behind, as well as a little boy who found his way back into the classroom. Apparently, unknowingly to me they had decided to lash out at me.

The boy was running around playing with Kalie and after a few moments of whispering, they asked me to play tag. As I refused he started putting his hand in my pants, I tried desperately to fight him off. I cried for help from Kalie, but she just sat watching quietly while ignoring my pleas for help. Once the class returned from recess, Kalie whispered around to all who would listen that I welcomed his advances. Finally, Kalie would announce in front of the whole class, "listen everybody we are gonna call her big nasty, ha, ha big nasty".

As she laughed and all her little followers concurred, I felt so hurt and embarrassed. Eventually, I despised daily the thought of even going to school and still quench even to this day when I hear anyone just mention that same horrible word even today. I started to feel as if I did something wrong and deserved this, as I could not figure out what I did wrong to God. But just as I could not take one more day of this ridicule, one student named Yolonda must have sensed my pain as she touched me on the shoulder and quietly handed me a piece of candy. I did not realize she was even in my classroom until that day. It was as though she appeared out of nowhere. Needless to say Yolonda and I became very good friends, she was as tall as Kalie, the bully, who was calling me names. Rolanda eventually gained the friendship all of Kalie's entourage leaving her furious.

Kalie kept on calling me names, but Yolonda grew tired of it and told her to, "shut-up". Kalie immediately asked her, "What do you have to do with it" as she raced toward her with built up jealousy. Yolonda did not like what Kalie was doing and they went at each other with a vengeance. So within moments the pushing started, and then the fight began. This was no doubt the fight of the century to me as fists were flying, and desks were pushed all over the place in the process. Ms. Swane ran out of the room screaming for help from the other teachers to help break up this fight in the classroom. They were not only hitting but scratching and pulling hair. Yolonda had a kind heart and knew what Kalie was doing was not right, as it appeared the teacher was not even there. As I looked back I almost feel it was a fight between good and evil. Yolonda was a true friend, and I knew deep down inside the very depths of my soul God still cared as he sent me a most needed guardian angel in the mist of my horrendous pain. I don't remember seeing Yolonda anymore or Kalie for the rest of the school year. I believe they moved them to another class with a teacher who could have more discipline over the classroom. Although they moved, some of the more loyal followers were left behind.

One morning not long afterwards my mother made me put on a dress that was a little too long and old fashioned, I begged her not to make me wear it but to no avail. That day as the some of the girls teased me saying my dress looked like my grandmothers', I felt betrayed once again. As I had to stand in front of the whole class to present my report, I went into a daze as I felt something running down my legs. The only thing I remembered was the teacher telling some students to get paper towels for the floor. As the teacher let me go home early that day, I was so distraught I ran all the way home while hating everything about that school. After that incident I did not recall Helen ever telling me what to wear to school again.

The rest of the school year was rather quiet, and it would be the last day of school before I would be stalked again. One of the last faithful followers told me, "I have been waiting all year to beat you up and I am going to get you today". She sat right across from my desk, and I had not realized how much she disliked me. I remember her telling me just a few weeks earlier, "Where did you get those shoes. I can't stand you". As they were the shoes my mother had purchased for my father's funeral.

I asked my best friend Wendy what was she going to do about the bullies and she whispered, "My mother told the teacher to let me out one hour early today". I immediately ran to the front of the classroom and whispered to the teacher, "I need to leave early today". Her first response was no. Then I proceeded to beg and pled with her to please let me leave like Wendy, I renounced again and again. Finally, she gave in and as I ran down the parking lot by the side of the classroom as the girl who threatened me earlier shouted from the second floor, "Where are going? I'm going to beat you up, so where do you think your going". I ran faster and faster until I could not see the school any more. I was so relieved the school year was over, and was quite surprised to hear teachers' had only a couple of fight's to breakup that afternoon.

✠ ⁓⁓ ⁓⁓ ⁓⁓ ⁓⁓ ⁓⁓ ⁓⁓ ⁓⁓ ✠

Precious pictures of my parents. Two of the most loving parents a child could ever hope for.

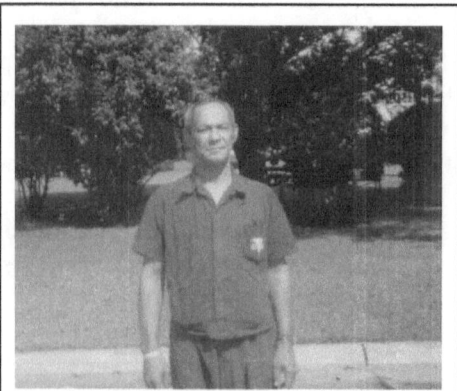

Picture of my father we took during one of his many stays while we were visiting him in the VA hospital.

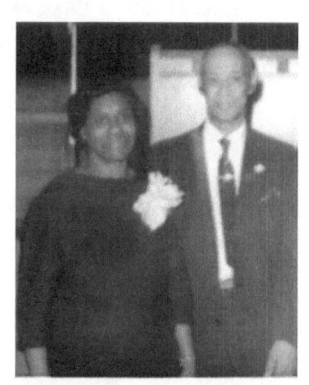

My mother and father pictured during my sisters first wedding in 1969 not long before he passed.

Chapter 2: Helen's Melancholy Memories

After Daddy's death Wendy and I would eventually loose contact with each other, as we would go to different schools. I sometimes wonder what my most dearest childhood best friend must be doing. Maybe a housewife with three children, or possibly a successful doctor or lawyer, but whatever she might be doing I hope she is well as I would often wish we had stayed in touch as adults, and continued to share our life experiences.

But my mother, Helen, would keep my mind preoccupied as she continually spoke of her pass experiences almost daily after my father passed. Sometimes the events spoken of were happy and most colorful with my father, but they were more often than not rather melancholic. She even spoke on subjects that occurred before her life with my Dad. Helen reminisced on things from deceased relatives to her life in California, as well as her first marriage before my father. My mother married her first husband, George, when she was only about eighteen and she mentioned he was a few years older than her. They further divorced a few years later, as Helen often spoke, "I am so glad I did not have any children by that no good lying George". Then she would just continue on talking about other things including her childhood experiences. She often mentioned attending the old Phyllis Wheatley High School and graduating at the top of her class.

℣ ℣ ℣ ℣ ℣ ℣ ℣ ℣ ℣ ℣ ℣ ℣

As family was the most important thing in life to my mother, it was also just as important to her mother Addie. It has further inevitably become important to me as well. It was the very fiber of life, and the core that gave Helen and her mother before her a reason for living each and everyday.

My mother spoke on how she born in Houston to the parents of Addie and Jim Phillips. Helen further advised that her grandfather was an American Indian, and her grandmother was of African American heritage.  They had a daughter, Addie, who was born in Huntsville, Texas.  Addie, my grandmother, probably moved to Houston in the early 1900's after her first husband passed away where she joined some of her relatives already living in the Houston area.  I recall as a very young child, visiting our cousin Emma.  My mother said it was her Uncle Willie's daughter.  Cousin Emma always called my mother and every once in a while we caught the bus from our second ward house to third ward to visit her.  We also had some other relatives of Addie's in town whom I did not have the privilege of meeting, although I did know all of my grandmother's children through my mother's spoken diary.

As my mother continued to inform us of our family tree, she said Addie's first marriage produced six children and the second marriage produced the last four children in which my mother was the youngest just as I.  Some of the siblings passed away before Addie.  I was not blessed to have known my grandmother but I feel as though I knew her very well, as my mother would reminisce even in the mist of her touch of memory lapses.  She often said how I reminded her so much of her mother.  Helen would even sometimes forget and call me mother, as I would sometimes give her herbs and make fresh vegetable soup just like her mother.  Addie had a full garden, which included herbs such as lots of mint tea and loved to make soup from the vegetables in her garden as well.  She was often thought of as the resident doctor of the neighborhood.  Addie treated all sorts of illness and often gave away items in her garden to strangers passing by.  Helen often spoke of people asking how much for the herbs, but Addie being a devout Christian would say,  "no charge".  Helen further mentioned how Addie's father was an American Indian, and he died before her birth.  So the old wives tale would decree that she could cure certain illnesses, because she never saw her father.  My mother told us how people would bring sick babies with thrush to my grandmother to blow into the baby's mouth, and the sickness would clear up.  As Addie had helped many people including my mother, who loved her so deeply she did not even want to see her die and preferred to precede her in death.  But Addie passed away before I was born in 1957.  She developed memory loss and often suffered with extreme confusion right before her death. Addie would talk of going home. Then she would take off walking and sometimes neighbors would call my mother saying Addie was with them, as they would help watch for her. It had gotten so bad at times my parents had to restrain her, as she would get up at night and start walking. They spent a large amount of time immediately prior to her death either watching or trying to find her. Eventually, Helen called the doctor and not long after that visit Addie would pass away. Helen felt the shot the doctor gave Addie speeded up her death, and often spoke of regretting the call she made to the doctor. She was very fond of her mother and always said, "There was not a better Christian in the world than my mother, oh how I loved my mother. I often prayed to God to let me die before her, because I knew I would not be able to get over her death. But when mother died there were so many people at the service. Some of the people there, I did not even know who they were. So many people loved her. She had a kind and giving heart and everyone who knew Mother, loved her. I can't even think of one bad thing to say about mother, and that's just how good of a person she was". Within all Helen's keepsakes lives sympathy cards, as well as telegrams of consolation for her mother's passing.

But Addie's death was preceded by five of her beloved children. Addie's daughter Elizabeth passed away first, she was called Lizzie for short. Helen spoke of how trusting her family was and thought of how her sister died not long after a neighbor prepared her dinner. In those days, the wake and funeral was at the home of the deceased. The next child to pass away was her son, Buddy, as almost everyone in the family had a nickname primarily because children were named after someone else already in the family. My mother did not remember much about my Uncle Buddy, Buddy died when she was young so she rarely spoke of him. Her brother Fred would be next to pass whom my mother named her firstborn after. He died young as well but Helen often spoke words of praise for her brother, "He would drop by mother's as often as possible, and when he arrived he would always cook for Addie. My brother Fred could make the best and fluffiest homemade biscuits in the world. That man could really cook, and every time he came by he would cook for mother."

The fourth child to precede Addie's death was Helen's sister, Velma, in about 1939. Velma sensed her death was near after returning home from the doctor's office the previous day. Helen never really knew what happened at the doctors' office, but felt it may have been related to her most untimely death. Helen further revealed one of her newborn babies had died. I remember Helen often quoted her mother saying after looking in the infant's face, "She has the face of an Angel. That baby is an Angel from heaven and she is not for this earth". The infant eventually passed away and I figured Velma probably found it very difficult to have another child, and I often thought how Velma could have possibly died from a badly done abortion. Also, Helen mentioned how back in those days abortions were done with coat hangers, and her death was preceded by a visit to the doctor, after which she could not stop bleeding. So I always thought it might have been an abortion, which went bad. But whatever the cause, the fact of the matter was her sister Velma passed most prematurely. And although Velma was married, she passionately pleaded with her mother, Addie, and Helen to please take care of her children. Addie would raise and keep the children together as promised along with my mother, Helen who would oversee the four children into adulthood as they thought of Helen as their second mother. Finally, on her deathbed and just moments before the end Velma stated, "I have a taste for some liver, Helen go tell mother to fix me some liver and onions". Shortly after eating Velma passed away. Then at the young age of fifteen, Helen was forced to assist her mother, Addie, with raising her sister's four young children with the youngest being only two years old. Velma left four children behind, the eldest, whom Helen often referred to as Junior, next was Florene. A second daughter, Hortense, and the youngest son was Paul. Helen and her mother struggled to raise four small children, and I am sure that they both did their very best. Helen's brother, Charles, and sister, Katie, did as much as expected considering they were young adults wanting to live their own lives. Helen always spoke of her mother and her siblings who had passed away much too soon, but now I would start to experience the tragedy of loosing loved one's at a very young age.

Before returning to Houston to care for her aging mother, Helen lived with her sister Mary for a few years in Oakland, California. But little did she know her sister Mary would pass away before her ailing mother. She was born January 8, 1909 as I read from the obituary in Helen's keepsakes. Mary wanted so much for Addie, Helen, and her deceased sister Velma's children to come live with her in California. She sent money for them to be able to come and visit. But they would never stay, Addie could not leave Houston and eventually in 1955 the fifth child to precede Addie in death was Mary. Helen often spoke, "If I had not left Oakland, maybe my sister Mary would still be alive". Mary died in her youthful forties, and Helen spoke of a the caesarian birth she had a years earlier, and against the doctors advise she had yet another child. Mary had three daughters. All of which died far too early deaths as well. Helen carried a lot of guilt feelings for the tragic events in her family. She loved her sister Mary very deeply just as she loved her mother, and all her family.

℣ ℣ ℣ ℣ ℣ ℣ ℣ ℣ ℣

The first death I recalled as a child was my mother's oldest sister, Aunt Berda, who was born in eighteen hundred and ninety six on the first day of June, which was the exact same day I was born. One year we celebrated our birthdays together, as I was so young I could barely remember. But I did recall the wonderful homemade ice cream Aunt Berda made, and having a good time playing in the park on the merry-go-round. Aunt Berda went to New Bethel Baptist Church along with my mother. I remember we loved her to bring that tasty smoked ham and sometimes fried chicken, as we would sit on the back pew awaiting her Sunday in-service snack. Aunt Berda would pass the food out during church, as we were deeply disappointed if she did not bring her leftovers to church. As we would sometimes munch while my mother would sing in the choir.

Helen loved to sing in the church choir. I was only about five or six years of age but I recall one song in particular she would lead, as I thought she would sing a bit nervously, "There is always somebody talking about me, trying to stop and block my progress most of ti~~~~~me. But the mean things they say don't make me feel bad, as I Got Friend they never thought I had, I got Jesus, and I kno~~~~w that's enough". As our one usher Sister Tennie Mae, always clapped enjoying the music as she stood at the door greeting everyone with a large smile. She wore the same ensemble every Sunday, which encompassed a white uniform, nurse cap, and white loafers. Sometimes she escorted me to the front row to sit as Helen sang in the choir. It was bad enough to miss out on the snacks, but then I would have to sit on the front row. I sometimes sat right next to her grandson Jose, whom everyone called Booboo for short as he always had a runny nose. He was a few years older as my small frame sat very low looking up, while he sniffled and never really wiped his runny-nose. If I was fortunate enough to sit on the back pew, Sister Strowder always sat right in front of us with her wide brim hat that concealed our most unorthodox but fulfilling behavior, as we sometimes left the house so early we often missed breakfast. And my dear Aunt Berda knew the right time to pass the snacks which was basically during the sermon, or when everyone was preoccupied and would not notice.

Afterwards I would always go to sleep immediately, as my sister Sophia would sometimes lay a handkerchief on her lap for me to nap during the sermon.

Aunt Berda would eventually stop attending church with us, and not long afterwards she would pass when I was no more than six years of age. What I recall mostly about Aunt Berda was how nice she dressed, as she most certainly did not look like a seventy-year-old lady. She wore those high-heeled pointed toe shoes like most of the church sisters. One of my young friends called them 'kill a roach in the corner shoes'.

She had three sons and one daughter. The eldest son Cornelius joined the Navy stationed in Hawaii, and my mother told me how Aunt Berda received a telegram one day. It advised that her son was hanged for some crime he committed while in the Navy. Aunt Berda felt he did not commit any crime and as he was a very handsome man, she felt his death might have been due to some jealous camaraderie. Her other son, Theodore, married and had about four children and moved his family to San Francisco. Before he passed away he often called or visited my mother, as they were not only almost the same age but were raised together and had a very close relationship. I now occasionally talk to his daughter, and she advised his other children are doing well, and a couple of his sons are currently in politics and law.

Berda's next son Leo passed in the 1970's, and her last son Raymond passed in 1990. Aunt Berda's youngest and only daughter, Ruby Lee, married Richard Williams and had two children Richard and Juliet. They named their son, Richard Cornelius after his father and deceased Uncle.

A few months before Aunt Berda's death, Berda decided she was going to live with us. I recall she was sleeping on the sofa one night, and her daughter Ruby Lee and her Husband Richard sat in our kitchen trying to devise a plan of how to get her home. Apparently she had developed memory problems just like her mother, Addie. Somehow Ruby Lee talked her into going home with them that next day. Not long after that episode, I recall Aunt Berda's passing. This was the beginning of many tragic childhood memories of my relatives passing. As my mother's people would appear to pass away and in between my Dad's side of the family would pass as well. Either we would just hear about a loss, or would attend a funeral one right after the other. As a child I just recall people seemed to be always dying, but my parents tried to shelter us as I only remember actually attending about a couple of the funerals. I soon began to learn it was not the beginning for my mother Helen, but merely another day filled with pass and continuing sorrow of premature dying.

Although I did not know Helen's second oldest sister, Willie, very well she born was in eighteen hundred and ninety eight and lived to be seventy-two years old, passing just about one year after Aunt Berda in 1970. Willie was named after her uncle, Addie's brother. I always felt he encouraged Addie to come to Houston after her first husband's death.

My Aunt Willie's husband was Reverend Author Gaines who passed in 1996 at the wonderful golden age of one hundred years old. The eldest son was named after his father, whom everyone called Sunny for short. They had five children, and Helen would sometime help baby-sit while Willie, whom they called Big Sister, worked in her beauty shop. Afterwards, Helen would help clean up the shop for Big Sister. Once while Helen baby sat her children, she accidentally dropped the youngest son Clyde right on the top of his head. Helen exclaimed how Big Sister raved, "Oh my Lord you have dropped my baby". As well as a few other choice words that were not quite as nice.

Helen was so proud of all her nieces and nephews' including Aunt Willie's or rather Big Sister's children Catherine, Herman, Faye Joyce, Sunny, and Clyde. The eldest son, Herman as well as his brother, Sunny both lived in third ward. When Herman fell sick with cancer Helen was devastated. Herman had taken ill before his mother passed in 1970. He lay sick not long after his mother's funeral service, finally Helen found out Herman was dying of cancer. The following Sunday we proceeded over to Herman's house immediately after church service. As we entered his house still dressed up for Sunday service, which seemed to be most fitting for what I thought was a mansion. It appeared to be a far cry from our small two-bedroom house, in second ward. We walked in and greeted his wife who took us through the living area, dining room, and then to the large beautiful mahogany stained bedroom.  But the house became most insignificant in comparison to my mother's dear nephews illness.  We later learned Helen was so upset as she stood over Herman lying in the bed covered with white linen.  In great shock and dismay Helen just blurted out,  "Herman, I did not know you were sick. Why in the Hell you did not tell me you were sick?"  Afterwards Helen broke down in tears, and would say very little over the next few days. She was really hurting over his sickness and his eventually his death. This was the beginning of what appeared to me as a lot of premature destruction and death of our family, as I would also later learn the distinctive correlation between nutrition and good health.

ᗡ ഇ ഇ ഇ ഇ ഇ ഇ ഇ ഇ ഇ ഇ ഇ

My mother's nephew, Herman, had purchased his house and owned some real estate in the area where Helen chose to send us to school.  I always felt one of the reasons why Helen identified with this area and chose to send us all the way across town to Woodson Elementary School, from second ward was partly because of Herman's influence.  As her loving nephew, Herman, would often stop by bringing clothes or something else he felt we might need. Helen was very close to her nieces and nephews, and further exhibited that closeness by eventually moving us all to a new neighborhood not far from where Herman's family was living.  It appeared to be a relatively quiet area, and I guest it was considered a really nice place to raise children.  As the area changed due to most of the people selling their larger homes in the Macgregor area, while other owners chose to rent the nearby smaller homes.  Only the rather affluent were able to purchase a home. The other side of third was mainly rent houses, where we eventually moved.  I found out a few years ago the area not far from where I lived was considered or referred to as 'The Bottoms'.  As we rented a house not far from the Gulf Freeway, I guess it was considered 'The Bottoms' as well. I knew we were poor, but I guess I did not realize there was separation of the classes in the third ward.

When we eventually moved to third ward, Aunt Katie, the oldest of Addie's last three children lived a few blocks from us. She was born in 1911 and had one son, Walter, and of course Aunt Katie had a nickname, 'Little Sister'. We would shorten the nickname even further calling her, Sister. As we were well within walking distance from her house when we moved to third ward, she would always call us to come pick up lots of freshly baked pastries. She baked tons of cupcakes, pies as well as a beautifully prepared dinner and decorated cake for each of our birthdays. She never missed baking on holidays either, until she feel prey to an infection in her foot. The infection started in her toe as doctors suggested removing the infected toe only, but against doctor's advice she refused surgery and the infection traveled to the leg. She eventually had her leg amputated at the thigh as Helen, Sophia, and Aunt Katie's son, Walter carried her forcibly to the hospital. As she lived four more years after that incident reaching the ripe age of eighty-three, and I still often felt she would have lived even longer. As I blamed myself for not checking on her like I normally would have, but I was so preoccupied since Helen's health began to worsen in 1996. She called and talked with Helen everyday until that time, and when she could not reach her or any of us she literally worried herself into a complete frenzy.

Aunt Katie, my Uncle Charles, and my mother Helen, respectively were the last three children all born into a second marriage of Addie Moses to Jim Phillips. My Uncle Charles was born in 1914 and as I viewed some of his older photo's, he was a nice-looking young man. I only new him in his latter years, we would eventually learn after his death that he married twice but ended up divorced each time. The first divorce was due to irreconcilable differences, as it stated in the divorce decree how she yelled and cursed him out repeatedly. But he loved sporting his cars and nice clothes. I remember his cars were always shiny, and although they were not brand new they were always spotless. What I remember most about my Uncle Charles, whom we called 'Brother', was the protectiveness and safeguarding of his nieces and nephews. He was always working and almost made retirement at his

Shell job, but started doing some security work. Although he was a good and honest man, he carried his security gun with him everywhere as he was a very unyielding man. I remember riding with him in his car and if someone was driving to slow, he would get so mad and start honking his horn and pointing. I was always so nervous around him. I guess it was mainly because he never talked very much and always exhibited a very serious demeanor. But I guess his serious behavior was due to his concern for maintaining our safety as wells as for himself. My Uncle passed exactly one year after his sister Katie in July 1997.

It was at Aunt Katie's funeral that I learned Uncle Author Gaines Senior, my Aunt Willie's husband had died only a few months before at the ripe age of one hundred. I learned he was still alert, living in the same house alone, and still driving until a few months before his death. This was no doubt a great inspiration to my psychic, as I would learn that my family could live long healthy lives. As most family's we lost contact and I mentioned to Faye Joyce, my late Aunt Willie's daughter, how I desired to plan a family reunion before Katie's death. But I guess I waited a little too long. After the funeral Faye Joyce and I decided we should still put together the reunion and we did. We had the reunion at her brother's, Sunny's house. I ordered the T-shirts with Addie's picture in the middle surrounded by all her children' names and birth dates. All of Helen's children and her late sister's children would attend including Aunt Berda's daughter's family, Aunt Willie's children, and Aunt Velma's grandchildren, and great grandchildren. Aunt Katie's son Walter', and Uncle Charles attended as we were able have the reunion before his death in 1997. I tried desperately to contact Helen's sister Mary's family in Oakland, but to no avail. As I researched through all of Helen's old photo's and papers for names. I was only able to find a couple of funeral programs with names, one of which Helen kept from her sister Mary's funeral in 1955 as well as her daughters in 1980. I proceeded to call Oakland's phone information from some of the names listed. After calling numerous residences, I still could not locate any of the Oakland born relatives. But the reunion went on as Helen was the life of the party, she exclaimed, "My Big Sister, Willie, was something else.  I use to go over to her beauty shop to get my hair done, but end up baby sitting and cleaning up.  One day while I was helping with Big Sister's children, Author Junior fell on his head and Willie screamed and swore at me for a while.  And look at him over there, see, that's what's wrong with him, he was dropped on that big head."  Everyone laughed as Helen kept us most amused by repeating her stories over and over.

ᴕᴕᴕᴕᴕᴕᴕᴕᴕᴕᴕᴕᴕᴕᴕᴕᴕᴕᴕᴕᴕ

Although the dying ceased for a while during my teenage to adult life, it would appear I should have been used to death as a part of life.  But I still felt overwhelming guilt along with the great sadness after my Aunt Katie's death.  If I had just cared for Helen from the onset of her sickness, maybe Sister and Brother would not have worried so much and would still be alive.  As I took my daily thirty-minute drive to work, I would cry the whole way asking God why.  I knew Katie was in good health, and so I continued to blame myself for her most untimely death.  Then after a few weeks passed, Sharon, Katie's daughter-in-law advised Katie had just walked out of the hospital a few days before she passed away.  Sharon further stated,  "Katie was in the hospital about a day, then against the doctor's advice she left with a bladder infection.  The doctor gave her a prescription but she refused to take the pills."  As I learned from Aunt Katie as well as Uncle Charles death certificates I inherited, that they both died of heart attacks.  I would later discover through my extensive reading that most elderly people die from heart attacks, which primarily stem from untreated bacterial infections.

I finally came to the realization that I could not continue dwelling on feelings of guilt any longer, but concentrate on providing adequate care for Helen.  I had to do what I had to do which was the right thing, and do it to the best of my abilities just as Helen did by helping raise her deceased sister' Velma's four children as a young teenager.  Helen often said, "Sister was too busy to help me, and mother raise my late sister Velma's children".  Although I am sure all Helen's siblings had good intentions, Helen became the four children's surrogate mother after Addie died.

Today all four of Velma's children have joined their mother in heaven. Helen often reminisced on how Junior died, the oldest of the four, who passed away first. Helen spoke very slowly and rather somberly about Junior as she reminisced, "I looked through the door and saw him lying on the table, and I know it was Junior. The pathologist had already cut his head and begun his procedure, and I started to scream, as they pushed me away from the door. I know that was Junior, I saw him, but the hospital would not let me in the room to see his face. They hurriedly pushed me back out of the room but I knew it was Junior. The hospital said he died from a blood clot in his head, but I knew how it happened. It was Zelda, the lady he lived with, and she was always fighting. She was so jealous of Junior, because he was so much younger than she was. He and Bella had a fight the week of his death, and I remember that she hit him over the head with something and he never recovered."

When Junior died in 1960, he was in the prime of his life. Helen was pregnant with me, and talked of how she just sat alone and cried. Maybe that's why I'm so easy to shed tears as well as a loner. This was another extremely hard episode in my mother's life, as she helped raise these small children into adulthood. Helen loved all of her sister's Velma's children like her own yet they all died much too young.

Florene was the second born child of Velma. Florene had one son, and Helen thought his late father had a very smart and foul mouth. I remember Helen saying, "He made me so angry one time that I told him someone is going to kill you one day about that no good foul mouth of yours". And Helen told us someone actually killed him by shooting him in the face. Florene eventually ended up with older man named Jack. In the mid 1960's Jack and Florene owned a tavern on Lyons Avenue in the fifth ward area where people could play pool, drink alcohol, and even gambled a little. Her son was over our house a lot until his mother's untimely death. I guest her murder had something to do with the gambling that night before, because in broad daylight a man walked in the bar and shot Jack in the back and Helen's dear niece, Florene. The bullet went straight through Florene's heart. Her husband Jack would later die at the hospital, but Florene died instantly. After we heard of the shooting, Helen rushed over immediately. I remember sadness while I sat in the taxicab outside as she pushed her way in yelling and crying, "I'm her Aunt, let me through, and let me through". I recall crowds of people standing around with the police trying to see what happened. I guest the police advised my mother to identify Florene, because I heard her crying hysterically. The next morning I recall Helen's picture in the paper while she held her hands over her face crying.

The one thing I remember most about my cousin's Florene visits was how she sat me on one knee and my sister, Sophia on the other. She would sing a cute little song about a cat and mouse running up a tree. I remember a big smile and a scar on her face as she shook us on her knee. Jack, her husband, would just sit on the sofa and eventually fall asleep, as she would always have to wake him when she was ready to leave. Her son who we called Little Paul came with her to visit us sometimes. He was a teenager at the time his mother was murdered and choose to live with one of Florene's acquaintances. We often felt her friend fought so hard to keep Florene's son merely for money. She would be able to receive some insurance benefits and possible government assistance. Helen learned years later that this woman was living with another lady whom was killed, and forced Little Paul to help drag the body out of the house where they eventually laid the body on railroad tracks. This was no doubt a horrible tragedy for a child to have to experience, as he would later become rather distance and estranged from the family.

Big Paul, the youngest child of Helen's deceased sister Velma only knew Helen as his mother as he was about two when his mother died. He loved Helen dearly and even confided in her even before he would marry his wife. Big Paul married Alice and had six girls and two boys. He would eventually develop a chronic heart condition. Doctors warned him if he did not change his eating habits, he might have to contemplate major heart surgery. Paul did very well for a few years, but by the age of fifty-seven Paul never recovered from his heart surgery. In

1994 not long after his death, Helen's health started to worsen. I believe my mother had taken as much as she possibly could, as her delicate arthritic condition did not even allow her to attend the funeral services.

Hortense, the third born child of Helen's sister Velma's was the last to pass away. She gave birth to her first child at the tender age of sixteen. A couple of years later Hortense met and married a gentleman named Boutee. As they decided to move to Dallas and wanted to take Hortense's two-year old baby daughter, Helen would not allow her to take the baby to Dallas. I am more than sure Helen help name the baby after Hortense's late mother, and since Hortense was rather young she still felt that duty to see after her late sister's children. That same attachment would cause Helen to raise and eventually adopt little Velma. After Hortense moved to Dallas, she had six more children with her husband. She eventually passed away at the age of sixty-two from a fatal caesurae. The doctors had taken her off the medication for a long while, but this last attack would prove fatal. After being off most medications for a year, everyone was shocked at her sudden and unexpected passing in 1995 not long after her brother's death in 1994. Again Helen sat in her wheelchair unable to attend the funeral service in Dallas.

~~ ~~ ~~ ~~ ~~ ~~ ~~ ~~ ~~ ~~ ~~ ~~ ~~ ~~

Hence, my mother continuously remained reminiscence after my father passed and vowed to never remarry, as she felt out of respect for her deceased husband and our father, her job was just to raise us. She further spoke of how Daddy did not have the privilege of going to school everyday, but rather grew up working in sugar cane fields. After his experiences in Jeanerette, Louisiana, Daddy felt the only way to make a good life for us was through a good education. This was something my Dad was robbed of by his own father, as it was an accepted circumstance for the family's to sustain their livelihood. Daddy knew the pain of missing your childhood and the cost of being deprived of a good education felt like, and refused relegate that same awful feeling to his children. Helen and Daddy wanted the best for their children, they yearned for a better life for us. As they spent much of their lives as humanly possibly to make that dream a reality.

My parents met a few weeks after Helen returned to Houston from Oakland. Helen was about twenty-five and Daddy was about thirty-two and my mother loved my father so much, I do not think words could describe her love for my father. Not long afterwards, my oldest brother Fred was born on June 12, 1946 in the house where Helen grew up on North Chartress Street in second ward. Fred was named after Helen's late brother. My parents sometimes tried to name their children after someone in the family they admired and deeply loved.

My mother and father had five children, including my cousin Hortense's baby girl, Velma, whom they adopted. Velma was born on March 26, 1951 at 1813 Bramble Street. This is the house that my Uncle Author Gaines married my parents in, and my oldest brother, Fred was born June 12, 1946. Also, their next three children would be born in the exact same house starting almost ten years later including myself. First, my brother Charles was born on February 4, 1956, whom my parents named after my Uncle Charles. Helen talked of how my brother Charles would crawl into the room every morning, where Addie used to sleep. Months after her death he would still look for my grandmother, Addie, as she passed around July 1957 a year and a few months after Charles was born. Charles, Sophia, and myself, the last three, were all born just about two years apart. Sophia was born May 1, 1958 and was named after my father's mother. I was born June 1, 1960 and to my knowledge was the only child not named after an existing relative.

The Bramble Street house is where I arrived from Jefferson Davis Hospital. Helen often said how Ben Taub used to be called Jefferson Davis and reminisced over most of her experiences there. She talked about how the nurses walked around looking for the Caucasian family, because of Fred's skin color. My mother further stated she had to yell for them to bring Fred to her, "Hey, Hey, What are you all doing running around the place with my baby? That is my damn baby, and bring him here right now." I, on the other hand was the most pleasurable experience as I rightfully claim as she advised, "You were the easiest child I gave birth too". Helen said I was so easy she did not know she had given birth. Needless to say my mother was very outspoken or rather just a slight tad bit vocal while my father was almost the exact opposite. He was more reserved and rather quiet, as he only voiced his opinion when needed. He appeared to always have something on his mind. I feel that I took after my father as well, because I thought more than I verbalized. I feel my Dad was a very deep and intelligent man, but lacked opportunities to achieve his desired greatness.

My father was born in Jeanerette Louisiana to Ophelia and Cecil Broussard. They named him Hilton Bernard Broussard on January 13, 1911. Although I believe there were about nine children born out this marriage only about six of them found their way to Houston Texas to my knowledge. Daddy spoke of his mother's long yellow hair. As both my great grandfather's were from France, most of my father's siblings either looked Caucasian or looked like my father, a light-skinned African-American who could not speak any English upon his arrival to Houston. It was around 1943, not long after his discharge from the army air force where he worked in a laborer capacity. Helen kept everything, which proved most beneficial to gain inside knowledge of the family history.

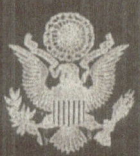

## Honorable Discharge
### from
## The Army of the United States

### TO ALL WHOM IT MAY CONCERN:

This is to Certify, That* HILTON B. BROUSSARD

† 38,204,525, Private, 358th Aviation Squadron, AAFES

THE ARMY OF THE UNITED STATES, as a TESTIMONIAL OF HONEST AND FAITHFUL SERVICE, is hereby HONORABLY DISCHARGED from the military service of the UNITED STATES by reason of ‡ ODD, 2nd Ind., Hq. Brooke Gen. Hosp., Ft. Sam Houston, Texas, dtd. 9 Sept/43.

Said HILTON B. BROUSSARD was born in Jeanerette, in the State of Louisiana When enlisted he was 21 6/12 years of age and by occupation a Porter. He had Brown eyes, Black hair, Colored complexion, and was 5 feet 6 inches in height.

Given under my hand at Brooke General Hospital, Fort Sam Houston, Texas this 14th day of September, one thousand nine hundred and forty-three.

Major, Medical Corps,
Executive Officer

See AR 345-470.

As the discharge paper reads: To Certify That Hilton B. Broussard 14th day of SEPTEMBER ONE THOUSAND NINE HUNDRED and FORTY-THREE, from United States Army, Hilton B. Broussard, private was honorably discharged from Fort Sam Houston on September 14, 1943.

Daddy initially lived with his sister Zelia who was one of the first siblings to move to Houston and the eldest sister. Helen often reminisced about an incident with herself and sister-in-law Zelia, while riding the city bus. The incident occurred during segregation and my mother was pregnant. A Caucasian gentleman stood up and tried to give Aunt Zelia his seat, as she looked Caucasian. Aunt Zelia then cleared the seat for Helen, and then proceeded to swear because no one attempted to offer a seat to my mother. As she stated, "I wonder how could everyone just sit and let a pregnant woman stand on her feet." Helen said she had never heard swear words put together quite like Zelia could do, it was a totally different language.

I remember my Uncle Wilfred very well, my father's oldest brother, as he died few years after my father. His medium-long blonde straight hair and bright baby blue eyes made him often mistaken as a Caucasian. But although Wilfred, Zelia, and some of my other relatives looked and shared more of the appearance of their French counterparts or relatives, they chose to live life acknowledging their African heritage. But if they had not made that choice, they would still be my relatives just as my French counterparts. Another one of my father's siblings was named Mondeveil, whom I did not have the pleasure of meeting. My mother said one of my father's brothers had dated a Caucasian lady, so I thought he might have lived and passed as Caucasian. I further recall a rather strange meeting of what appeared to be with an older Caucasian man. After a downtown grocery store trip one afternoon, my parents and myself were waiting for bus. While waiting, this man approached us, who had straight blond hair. As I was about five years old or so, I looked in freight from his scruffy appearance. He appeared unshaven and a bit soiled as I was so afraid he would hurt me, but even odder he started trying to hand me a dime. Thus, I would merely let it drop to the ground being totally terrified of this stranger. My mother exclaimed, "It's okay you can take the money". He would try to give me the coin once more only to watch it roll down the sidewalk once again. As he would pick it up again and laugh, "That's okay, Mama you take it".

Helen would reply, "Thanks", and as he walked away my mother would renounce once again, "You were right Nanette, never take money from strangers. But since we were with you, it was all right". Although I did not know who that man was, and I don't think he was even related to us. But I imagine in my yearning to visualize all my father's siblings I would let my imagination runaway, as I later thought he resembled some of my relatives. Trying to fill the void of the unknown I did know one thing for sure, and that was I loved my relatives no matter what their appearance or status or background. Helen later revealed Mondeveil died of lung cancer or rather tuberculosis, as there was not a cure during 1950's or 60's.

I further did not know my father's brother Ameil, as I do not know if he even traveled to Houston. Besides the generally intolerable working conditions and low share cropping compensation, I tend to think there was more to my father's families past. Maybe another reason why Ameil did not make it to Houston or others left and did not desire to return. My brother thought my father mentioned he died accidentally. I guess we can only imagine and wonder about all the gory details and the why's as they caned sugar in the swamps of Louisiana. As I imagine four small boys Mondeveil, Ameil, my father Hilton, and Oneal trying to cut sugar cane with huge machete knives larger than their tiny bodies. Barely or rather unable to see in front of their little faces over the tall stalks and other workers, I guess it was a miracle any of them survived the experience.

Another sibling, Olivia moved to Beaumont and married as I did not know her, but I did know her children James, Alice, and Morris. Although I did have the privilege of meeting Olivia's husband whom everyone called Babe for short. As I could barely recall the visits, because I was no more than possibly five or six years old at the time. Even though Olivia, my father sister had passed, her husband, Babe would continue to visit my father with his two sons Morris and James, as well as James wife, Beatrice. As Beatrice would always bring some really strong Community coffee, and those wonderful stage plank ginger pastries, which was once again one of the few items I loved to eat as a little girl.

I recall sometimes visiting my father's youngest brother, uncle Oneal, a very handsome man who lived alone in a small one-bedroom apartment. A few years after Daddy passed, he was found dead in his apartment from a fatal blow to the head and his apartment was ram-sacked. My mother thought someone probably followed him home and waited to rob him as he lived alone. The youngest sibling was Aunt Ovella who moved to Houston as well. While Aunt Ovella never had children, she did marry and raise two of her niece's children. The children were her sister Zelia's granddaughter, and her brother Wilfred's grandson.

My father said Cecil had or rather fathered about thirteen children. I met one of my father's half sister's, Stella. Stella would come and visit us every Friday evening once we moved to third ward. She lived a few blocks from our house on Palmer Street. As she would stay until her and my Dad would get into a heated argument. I don't remember what the arguments were about, but I do recall my father's teasing and laughing at her, and Stella saying all types of swear words. Then she would storm out yelling, "I ain't never coming back to this house no more". But she always returned until my father's most untimely death.

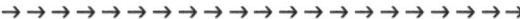

Recently I planned my first visit to Jeanerette, Louisiana with my cousin, Joseph whose mother is my first cousin, Rose. Rose along with all her brothers and sisters were born in Jeanerette to my father's oldest brother Wilfred, and his first wife Sylvina. But oddly enough as we were planning, that Memorial Day weekend my first cousin Rose passed away. We later learned her ninety-eight year old mother, Sylvina, lay in a recovery center after recently experiencing a severe stroke.

I decided to attend the service and asked my older brother Fred go with me, as he knew Rose very well. Rose had moved to Houston and later moved to Maryland to live with her daughter, Doris, until her battle with cancer overcame her. The arrangements had been previously made for her burial in Jeanerette. As we returned from the gravesite to my first cousins home, we noticed rows and rows of what my brother thought was rice. After asking my relatives what was growing on their land, they advised they lease out the property and receive monthly payments for growing sugar cane. How ironic as I learned it was all sugar cane, nothing but sugar cane for miles and miles. Some of the exact same fields my father and his siblings would walk cutting by hand for hours to no end as little boys and into their adulthood, until they decided to move. Downtown Jeanerette appeared to resemble the early 1900's, as it was a visit from the past and no doubt a bittersweet experience. Although my brother liked the town of Jeanerette, I could not help but reminisce on my father's words of having to quit school to help cut sugar cane. I continued to feel an eerie almost haunting feeling the whole way there and back. As I saw sugar cane growing for miles and miles all over Louisiana, my oldest brother, Fred, finally reiterated how my father and his brothers had to cut the cane with mushede knives. Although I enjoyed visiting the place my father was born and meeting the relatives and their neighbors, it would be months before I felt some relief from the trip. It was as though I could feel the haunting spirits of sadness from my father's past amidst a seemingly peaceful town.

ααααααααααααααααα

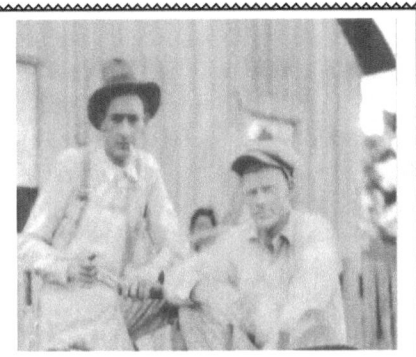

My Uncles Wilfred and Oneal are pictured at the sugar mill around the mid 1930's.

I took some old photos that my father had kept from his youth growing up in Louisiana along on our somber visit. I always wondered who some of the people actually were on the photos. As I showed everyone the pictures from my father's collection, the first picture was of my uncle Wilfred and one of the younger brothers, as we were trying to figure out which one.

Then my cousin Rose first husband, who was about eighty-three looked at the picture and said, "Ooh that's Oneal. We use to fight everyday and I would run home", as we all just laughed. I continued to show the pictures to the elder neighbors, but they were never able to figure out who the other two strangers were on the picture. I guess someone decided to take a photo of my Uncles and two other workers, as they worked the fields that day. Little did that person know it would become my father's treasure, and now mine.

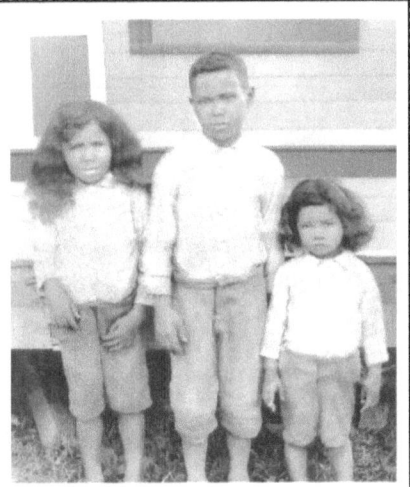

My father, Hilton, pictured in center with a fresh haircut, and my uncles pictured on each side. Photo taken around 1920.

The next picture I showed was a childhood photo with my father in the middle, who had just gotten a haircut along with uncle Oneal who was the youngest boy and possibly Uncle Ameil. As my father had just gotten a haircut, he and my uncle Wilfred would always argue about who stood nice and clean-cut in the middle. As we all could tell it was my father including uncle Wilfred, but I think they got their kicks out of teasing each other. Nevertheless looking at the three boys on the picture, I could only image what deep dark secrets lurked in my father's childhood. My father never really talked about Ameil, but I believe he was pictured next to my father just a few inches shorter, and on the other side of my father was Uncle Oneal. They looked solemnly sad on the picture, as all the boys had to quit school to cut sugar cane. I am sure it was a very dangerous experience with several small children in the field at once, and I can only image if maybe something tragically happened to one of the boys. But whatever happened in Jeanerette I did know my father as well as the rest of his siblings left Jeanerette for a better life, and I had no doubt from that day on he made a wise decision at that time. He wanted to make a better living and although he was not able to see all aspects of a better life, he did experience some form of relief if only to receive similar wage compensation by comparison. But the tradeoff was worth it, if my father felt some solemn peace from those most haunting sugar cane fields.

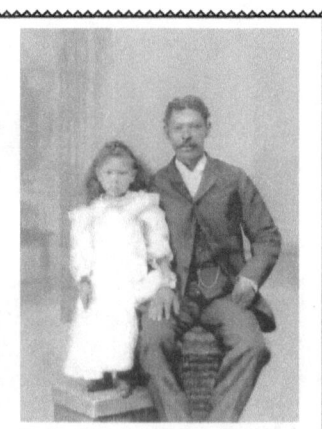

Early 1900's Formal Portrait of my grandfather Cecil and one of my Aunts.

I also had a picture of my Dad's father Cecil and one of my Aunt's. I found out from the restoration studio that this picture was taken in a studio with a cloth background.

We had further kept the original frame and I was saddened as it had gotten loss a few years ago, but the lady that was restoring my picture would ask, "Did you inherit that watch". As I looked closer at the picture I noticed Cecil had a pocket watch dangling down as I could only imagine what it might be worth today. Then I thought back as I recalled seeing a similar watch in my father things years ago, but as I looked at the picture again I was more joyous that my father was so sentimental and thoughtful. My father brought these keepsakes all the way from Jeanerette, and kept them safe for all these years. The photos were further confirmation that family was no doubt worth much more than riches, and these *pictures were in fact the true treasures.*

It was the last picture shown of one of my Aunt's pictured with my grandfather, I could only imagine it was my Aunt Ovella, the youngest one of all the siblings. My grandfather, Cecil, who caned sugar as a sharecropper, in the early 1900's until his untimely death around 1926. My father spoke of how they caned sugar and owned a sugar mill in Jeanerette in the early 1900's.

He further spoke of his mother with long yellow hair, and how one his grandmother's were born in Jamaica while his grandfather's on both sides were Frenchmen. I could only imagine one of his grandmothers was from African descent, and possibly traveled from Jamaica with some inspiring hope to the Louisiana swamps. My father said my great grandfathers on both sides were from France as I could tell by the most precise French my father spoke. By the time I was born, I believe Daddy had forgot almost all of his native language of French as he only spoke a few words from time to time. As I desire to trace as far back to Jamaica or Africa or even France if at all possibly. Although I know my father's immediate relatives, I still long to find and trace my family tree. The only other ancestry information I have besides my grandparents were Aunt Me, and Aunt My whom my father advised had moved to New Orleans. As these names were probably nicknames or expressions of my father's comical uniqueness, that further leaves a search from the New Orleans origin relatively futile. But I am sure some of my relatives probably choose to live separate only recognizing their Caucasian heritage, to avoid the unwarranted prejudice. Now it would appear without any shadow of a doubt that I would have a long, and hard task of even researching our immediate family tree with so little pertinent information.

There was also a strong possibility my great grandmother was one of the supposedly freed Caribbean slaves of the 1870's, and choose to stay with my French born great grandfather. As I sometimes wonder what part of France or who are my French ancestors. I further imagine a Jamaican lady around that old plantation house, as it appears most beautiful and spacious. As she looks out in the yard while the children run around playing and laughing. But then I see another most disturbing picture of my great-grand mother laboring in the sugar cane fields. A beautiful dark skinned lady who's expecting yet another child, while she labors beside her other children. As she would merely fall each time from overexertion and premature labor pains. Whatever truths the dark past may reveal, I would like to know all the true images of my ancestors. But for now I am happy with what I do know about the past, which is quite disheartening at times but mostly enlightening. As one learns how not to repeat the past mistakes, in which my father knew so very well.

My father told us he stopped attending school after third grade because of his father Cecil's demands, "You don't have time to go to school. We need you to help work". They had to start working in the fields at a very young age to help make a living for the family, or rather for mere survival. My brother, Charles recently shared with me some of my fathers experiences growing up in Louisiana. My father confided in my brother a lot in his young life, as my father passed when my brother was only fifteen. My father talked of how he would ride his horse from their home in Jeanerette to New Orleans. He would pick up the bananas that would fall off the boats as they unloaded, and would eat so many bananas that he made himself sick. My brother further told me how Daddy said our grandfather, Cecil passed, as it seemed rather strange that I suffered with the exact same ailment as a teenager. He told me how my Father at the young age of fifteen, rode his horse as fast as he could into town to get the doctor after Cecil had taken ill. But by the time he returned with the doctor, his father had died from a ruptured appendix and coincidentally I had my appendix removed as a teenage.  Daddy often reminisced on how everyone came and just took furniture, and other belongings from their house after his father passed. I heard one of our relatives mention Cecil had a gambling problem, but I feel they probably took valuables to pay off the unreasonable debts incurred by share cropping.

My father taught himself how to read and write, as he read very well and although his handwriting was not perfect it was quite legible. This enabled him to enroll in Texas Southern University's Vocational School, after his discharge from the Army Air Force.  I still recall his shoe repair equipment, and sometimes I even remember hearing him hammering while fixing a shoe heal from time to time.  I guess this was all the college was able to offer him considering his third grade education level.  As I read through his 1948 catalog I saw my fathers name printed in the following manner under the graduate register, 'Broussard, Hilton: Voc.', which meant he was a recent graduate from TSU's Vocational School.  I also noticed the name Wilfred Broussard right under my father's, which could only mean that my uncle decided to attend the college as well.  It would be only a few months after my oldest brother Fred was born that my father enrolled in college.  It reminded me of my own life and how my son Joseph inspired me to return to college. I still have my father's college catalog from 1948-1949, and as I read through the catalog I found the College did not offer a G.E.D. Curriculum during that time.  The only curriculum the college made eligible for my father was the Vocational School, as it required graduation from an accredited high school with an exception for veterans. The school was founded in 1927 and shared the Jack Yates High School building, and in 1945 bought a 53-acre campus site on Cleburne.  This would be the exact same college I would attend more than thirty years later, as I entered college upon my graduation in September 1978.  Subsequently my father attended his classes on the relatively newly opened campus. Although my father did not have very much of an education which limited his opportunities, he did have a deep-rooted desire for all his children as well as a great dream that we would one day finish high school and be able to attend any school of higher education. He knew because of his lack of education, his choices were limited, but as he loved us very deeply and desired us to have the chance he did not or could not have. I believe his father, Cecil, literally had to rob him and his siblings of that chance in order to survive. My father, his siblings, as well as his father, Cecil before him knew first hand the evils of being poor as I grew more tolerant of understanding their pass decisions and why most of them turned to alcohol for a bit of piece and comfort in the mist of inequitable circumstances.

My father knew with an education, one could succeed and have a better quality of life. As my father tried desperately everything within his power to give us that better life, and in an effort to achieve that desire I recall how my father had held on to some old coins. It was buffalo nickels, pennies, and a few other old coins. I believe some of the coins were acquired from his father Cecil as well as my brother, Fred, advised he and a friend were playing in the backyard and found an old well. My father was then able to retrieve the coins from the well, and added them to his collection. He held on to them as he new they would be worth the effort. But to our dismay one of my mother's relative's son, who we later learned had a drug habit lifted the jar of coins out of my father's dresser drawer. My father was devastated, as he knew this was his last hope for providing a good and descent life for his family. Not long before the coins were stolen, I recall my father and mother discussing their plans of buying a house. As I also learned they were trying to save for my older sister's college education. So I always felt that my father wanted to eventually sell the coins and purchase a house for us, or use it to help with our college education. That was no doubt one of the most single devastating events in my parent's life.

After all we were already poor, and having the small treasures swept from under you does take its toll on a family. Also I guest being born in the 60's when it was still a lot of unfortunate and blatant racism did not help matters, but through it all there were some very memorable times. I felt very fortunate to be raised by good people where although there were some negative events, I did have positive circumstances surrounding my childhood.  I had very good parents, teachers, preachers, aunts and uncles, and of course we were raised to put our hopes and dreams in nothing less than God and his everlasting greatness.  For the greatest gifts would ultimately come from the God, the father and Savior Jesus Christ in heaven.  We were taught that if you trust in God, you could accomplish anything that you put your mind to as you work diligently toward achieving that goal.

Chapter 3: Life After Death 'The Widowed and Fatherless'

Between the reminiscing on the past, my mother loved to speak well of all her children to everyone. She loved to brag about us, and eventually gained attention from Charles's forth grade teacher. Helen spent an enormous amount of time talking about his straight A's, and how ingenious he was. Charles's forth grade teacher realized it as well, and became very involved in our lives after my father passed in March of 1971. Helen told Mrs. Greer how Daddy felt finishing school was most important, and how it was his primary dream for all of us. Not long after Daddy died Mrs. Greer and her colleague, Mrs. Mathews, came to visit and kindly bestowed upon us some clothes and food. At the same time Mrs. Greer made a point to ask all of us what we wanted to be when we grew up. I don't recall what my siblings said, but I exclaimed, "I want to be a doctor". After Daddy had just died from a massive heart, I wanted to do everything I could to prevent this pain from happening to others. I knew whatever profession I would choose, it would no doubt be one to help others.

I can remember on one occasion Mrs. Greer inviting us over for Christmas. She had a beautiful three-bedroom house, with a two-car garage. I remember seeing the most beautifully decorated Christmas tree, it was such a big tree to befall a poor little girl from the so termed lowly second and third wards. As it nearly touched the ceiling along with lots of presents underneath, I recall thinking they must be extremely rich people. I still have the picture of my brother Charles as well as my sister Sophia, and myself dressed up so nicely next to the beautiful tree. Helen always dressed us so nicely with our mostly charitable clothes and neatly combed hair that, you could not tell how poor we really were. The following visit we spent the whole day, and she gave my sister Sophia and I each a doll. I recall Sophia wanted me to sit still all day like Helen had told us to. But I being a couple of years younger wanted to play. Mrs. Greer let us sit outside as her husband peddled around the yard. She had two teenage children of her own, Gary and Linda. We only saw them a couple of times, but they appeared to be just as nice as their mother. These teachers and their family's were very inspirational in our lives, as they were one of the first role models in my life to instill a determination of attending college and ultimately viewing my future in a most positive light.

Mrs. Greer requested I stop by her classroom every morning before class, as she opened her purse and handed me a dime for ice cream. I loved that treat since my parents were unable to afford such things. I recall one day mentioning to Helen what Mrs. Greer was doing, and she told me to stop going by her room. Even though I tried to tell Helen that Mrs. Greer insisted I come by every morning, but as she refused to reason. My mother did not want me becoming a burden or taking advantage of the teacher's kindness. After Mrs. Greer missed me coming by her room she asked, "Where have you been I missed you?" As I just shrugged my shoulders and she gave me a hug and said, " I miss you. So you just come on by whenever you wish." At the time, I did not understand why my mother said to stop receiving the money, as it appeared to be yet a small glimmer of hope from some new friends gained after a tragic loss of my father. So my regular teacher tried to make me drink milk after not having enough money for ice cream, but the first day it was sour and the lunchroom let me trade it for an ice cream. The next time it did not taste right once again, and seeing how they were gracious enough to trade it for ice cream before, I thought they could trade it again. But the cafeteria lady was not so understanding, as this large lady clinched her teeth saying, "You better get your but back that table and drink that milk, and bit not come in here again." I scurried out of the lunch line in shear fright and never drank again.

I recall staying up most nights being tragically frightened of the dark, and felt so unsafe. Daddy was not around anymore to walk the house during the night checking on us, so I felt we could not make it without him. Fearing someone or something would surely take my mother away or hurt us. I was so fearful that Helen, Sophia, and myself slept in the same bed, except for Charles. He slept in the back bedroom. One night I remember seeing a shadow in my mother's bedroom door, and I frantically awoke my mother. I woke her up quite often shaking, tossing, and turning, and this night she pulled me right under her arm very tightly. That night I felt less fearful, and was able to obtain a little rest.

My brother Charles appeared to have dealt with my father's death rather inwardly. Charles was the oldest of the last three of us, and he had just made fifteen. At that time neither he nor any of us decided to keep up Daddy's garden, as we were all rather young. Even though we knew Daddy still kept a garden, after we moved to the Palmer Street house. But I think we all felt it was much too painful to continue, as it was a gentle reminder of our loss. Charles spent a lot of time in the unattached garage located at back of the house. There was a fenced yard with a sidewalk leading to the front of the garage and another door to the side. Although we did not have a car, we were about the only boxcar house in that neighborhood with a dining room and a garage. In the two-car garage we stored lots of odds and ends including some pieces of wood. Somehow my brother started putting the odds and ends together and before long he was building things. I suppose for his healing from my father's death, he would poor his heart into it. The first item I recall Charles build was a picnic slash ping-pong table. We had loads of fun all day long as we all played ping-pong, and we became quite good at the game. Then he decided to build a couple of benches to go with the table. They appeared to look very well built and went well with the table, until one Saturday afternoon. My mother decided to sit on the side of one of the benches, within a moment the other side went fleeing straight up in the air. As the bench was very unstable my mother rolled to the ground while reaching in the air. Once we learned she was not hurt, we all laughed so hard we could hardly breathe. Afterwards my brother redid the benches by adding boards across the bottom for anchors. Needless to say my mother did not test the new benches, but opted to sit on the back concrete porch instead.

In between the building and back yard catastrophes, Helen ran into hard times caring for us as my father's VA pension was discontinued. We were then put in contact with a social worker who, had good intentions and attempted to help us. She told my mother she could get food vouchers and medical care, as she would exclaim, "We can even make you a dental appointment for your little one." I cannot figure out to this day why she felt I needed a dentist, although I am sure she meant well. But neither Charles nor my sister Sophia went to the dentist, as it was just myself. I still remember that most unmemorable day very well. They drilled and drilled as well as they did not administer enough novocain. So once again this was yet another total travesty, as my poor mother did even know what was happening. It was a brand new clinic just built on the southeast side with young dentists about the same age as the social worker. I guess they needed some business, but it was not worth the cost. They advised Helen I had eight cavities, all in my molars. Looking back on the experience I don't feel I needed quite that much dental work as I barely ate any food, and was not in any pain. Today I can honestly say as I deal with having these amalgams or silver fillings replaced by root canals and caps, that this was a big mistake. Furthermore, I later learned this material contained largely mercury. High mercury and aluminum toxicity has been linked to brain disorders including Alzheimer's, and various other sicknesses and disease as it seeps into your bloodstream. Although this particular material is no longer used, I still request tooth colored fillings and precious metals only for caps when visiting the dentist just as a precaution.

Although this was a horrible experience, I do recall other more pleasant experiences after my father's death. One Sunday afternoon while the pastor and his family were leaving the church located directly across the street, they decided to stop by our house. They knew our father had recently passed, so we thought they were merely coming by to render condolences. But to our amazement, they left us an offering. We could not believe people we did not even know left us money. Helen told us how my father often said that we would do much better without him, but I guess that was not exactly the case as we still depended on the charity of others. Not long after we received the offering from the pastor and his family, we decided to visit this church, which was named after St. Paul. My older sister Velma was the first to visit and one Sunday as I was not getting ready fast enough, she left without me.  As I walked down the long isle of the church, looking from side to side in my bright yellow ruffled dress Mrs. Bell from second ward had given to me, I finally heard Velma's voice. "Nanette, Nanette over here," she called slightly raising up from her seat, while motioning for me to come over. By summer we had all joined Saint Paul Church. Velma my oldest sister, had married two years ago and my father baby sat for her until he died. But she would divorce not long after we buried my father.  Velma decided to continue attending our old church in second ward, New Bethel Baptist.   Fred, my oldest brother married before Daddy died as well, not long after he returned from the marines as he, his wife, and their three sons attended St. Nicholas Catholic Church.

So that summer after Daddy passed Charles, fifteen years old, Sophia, thirteen, and myself almost eleven, attended vacation bible school at St. Paul.  Needless to say we were active and stayed at the top of our classes.  Once I recall the Pastor announcing from the pulpit to the entire congregation how smart Sister Helen Broussard's children were, and how everyone should be more like us.  Everyone also knew not to mess with Sister Broussard's children as she would always say, "I would die for anyone of my children".

Not long after we joined St. Paul, Helen worked with the mission while I joined the usher board. Sophia joined the choir and to our amazement sang very well, although I don't think she felt she was a good singer.  Charles joined the choir also, and only sang when they needed the baritones. We also participated in the usual Christmas and Easter plays.  Charles played Jesus one year, and everyone was shocked that he did not take the time to memorize his lines, as our once straight 'A' genius started to drift away from the church and school.  As my mother would loose the battle for awhile to his experimentation with drugs which eventually would lead to his hospitalization within two years. My fifteen year old brother took my father's passing the hardest of us all, as I eventually would realize exactly how very close he and my father actually were.

Helen would eventually become the church treasurer and the secretary, which handled all the church's business affairs such as banking and bookkeeping.

Members in the church would say nice things about us as well. One of the church members, Sister Moore bought my sister Sophia and I two beautiful dresses. She actually joined St. Paul not long after we did, as I believe God sent her to become our guardian angel. Bringing us clothes and food as her husband would often go fishing. I also had a very dear cousin, Paul, who would go out on his boat as well so we had lots of fish and sometimes even crabs for our Cajun gumbo. My father had previously showed my mother how to make a wonderful Louisiana gumbo rue. Moreover between the church folk and other good people helping us, we came to know the importance of what friends really meant very early on.

&#x2767;&#x2767;&#x2767;&#x2767;&#x2767;&#x2767;&#x2767;&#x2767;&#x2767;&#x2767;&#x2767;&#x2767;&#x2767;&#x2767;&#x2767;&#x2767;&#x2767;&#x2767;&#x2767;

One night during one of the Sunday night musicals at the church, I felt my first glimpse of a crush at the tender age of eleven. Our pastor always invited a few visiting churches. Rev. Coles from a church a few blocks away often hosted our Church anniversary that was synonymous for dressing old fashioned, and eating lots of barbeque as well. I recall on our most esteemed occasion of dressing old fashion we would wear ankle length cotton checkered and paisley pattern dresses with large sashes tied in back. Also we had beautiful large matching bonnets that a couple of church members made, while the guys wore overalls and of course cotton shirts.

But this night I noted a new visiting church for this particular musical. Rev. Coles preached as usual and as he got lost in the spirit he would first throw his handkerchief in the air and then catch it. Then he would stretch out his long legs and step over the banister of the pulpit as he shouted and strutted from one side of the church to the other. After the invigorating sermon we would have our musicians play almost till midnight. But there was a new visiting church that in fact were relatives of a couple our deacons, and lived close to our Pastor on the south side of town. This part of town was what I thought to be a step above our meager neighborhood, but all my attention was focused on this adorable medium blond little boy singing and dressed quite nice. He was about my age and sang with his brothers as they were all dressed alike in these cute pink shirts with white collars, white ties, white slacks, and with matching white shoes of course. The church loved the boys, and was ecstatic as they sung, "You're on the Right Road Now". As well as "Jesus Said He Would Fix It". I was pretty taken away with the lead singer, Sylvester. I could not wait to go to the back of the church and see him as I talked one of the girls into introducing us. As I walked to the back of the church, I was so nervous I felt my stomach turn. We just mainly looked at each other rather than talking, but he did ask for my phone number. After his first call I asked for his number, as I thought Helen would not approve. I was so afraid that Helen would find out that I just hurriedly hung up the phone. He would continue to call me for the next few years asking if my mother would let me date yet, but the answer was still the same. Finally, we lost contact until I was about twenty-one. He seemed like a nice young man and tried to make a go at the relationship again, but at that time I was too preoccupied or rather confused to make any logical decisions on real love. Then about another twenty years later, we met again but this time he was engaged.

As sometimes infatuation turns into real love and last a lifetime, but more often than not the sad truth is so many of us may miss out on the real wonderment of our true love.

ଛଡ ଛଡ ଛଡ ଛଡ ଛଡ ଛଡ ଛଡ ଛଡ ଛଡ ଛଡ ଛଡ ଛଡ ଛଡ ଛଡ ଛଡ ଛଡ ଛଡ ଛଡ ଛଡ

We stayed pretty busy after we joined the church across the street, I felt it helped us all cope with the loss of my father. Between the fish fry's and barbecue dinners we would help the church put together and sell, we barely had time to think. One Monday night I decided not to

attend usher board meeting as Charles attended alone.  Sophia and I
stayed at home and fell asleep in the back bedroom
while Helen had went to sleep in the front living room.  Helen mainly
slept in the living room chair as she started this routine right after Daddy
was diagnosed with heart disease.  That night when Charles returned
home to the dark backyard, he found it difficult to open the gate.  He
pushed the gate open with all his strength, as something lay behind it.
As he walked he started to step large puddles of what he called a thick
gooey liquid.  As he eventually wiped his feet and made his way into the
house to turn on the outside lights, he found our dog, Sergeant, lying
lifeless next to the fence.  As we tried to make sense of yet another tragic
event, Sophia's guard mother, a Spanish lady who lived across the street
from us in second ward advised,  "Whenever an animal is killed, he has
taken the place of the human being's tragic and violently death."  Helen
said it was someone after one of her girls, referring to Sophia and myself.
I knew she was probably right, because I always felt a very deep fear in
that house and this incident only made matters worst.

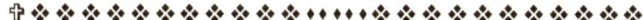

Church life appeared a bit better than school life, after my father
passed.  In sixth grade I was bused to a new school.  It appeared to be a
nice large school, as we loved play on swings and bars.  We also played
baseball and Hector one of my classmates would always hit the ball far
across the school's fence, and into the yards across the street.  Then one
day while in the outfield Hector hit one hard and fast, as it landed right in
my eye.  I whaled in pain from the hit, and the teacher told someone to
put some ice on it.  I was guided with my hand over my eyes to the
classroom still crying.  As my vision became quite blurred for a while, as
I believe this incident probably help contribute to my partial stigmatism
today.  I didn't even go to the school's nurse office, as my mother was
shocked to find out what happened that evening.  I had the same male

teacher the whole year, and his daily method entailed speaking only about race and the KKK. I thought this must be a conspiracy, since my fifth grade teacher had done almost the very same thing. But he talked about it daily, I guess he got away with it because he never tested us nor did have requirements except that we copy different parts of book. It was a total travesty. He was a lawyer by profession and always passed out his business cards to us.

Recess was the only high point of our mostly depressing day as I had made two good friends who were Spanish, Bianca and Marie. They loved to play but sometimes they played a little rough. I think they were trying to get revenge for another girl who had been bossing them around. Rosalinda was taller than the rest of kids and thrived on pushing them around. Until one day after watching me befriend the girls, she decided to change her wicked ways. I guess she envied my friendship with the girls, and I can't blame her as we did have loads of fun. We ran and played, while laughing loudly as we chased one another playing tag. After a few weeks, they stop hanging around me and became buddies with Rosalinda, as I am sure it was an offer they could not refuse.

৯৹ ৯৹ ৯৹ ৯৹ ৯৹ ৯৹ ৯৹ ৯৹ ৯৹ ৯৹ ৯৹

Middle school was the growing years full of dreams of the fu the beginning of feelings of love and romance. During seventh grade still very shy around people, and most especially the boys. As some kids invited me to different events such as picnics in the park, but as I knew Helen would probably say no, I did not even bother to ask. But on one occasion my friends told me how they played spin the bottle, and one of my friends advised how she had several kisses from cute guys. I remember one boy in particular named Paul. His last name was the same as mine, but we were not related, as I knew of. Everyone would ask us if we were related, but I was so glad to say no. He had a big soft neatly shaped medium blonde Afro, and was the best looking and coolest guy in the school I thought. I remember every time he walked into the classroom his fro would bounce just a little, almost just like my stomach when I saw him. But I believe my stomach bounced a lot more as it would literally turn over with mere excitement. As I had never felt that way since I met Sylvester, and so I knew I was head over heels in love. We talked often, and one day after walking me to the bus stop he asked if he could call me. Once again I told another new friend, that my mother did not let me receive calls from boys. That next school year Paul was not at school, I would never know what happened to him as I missed my dear friend very much.

That same year I thought I would make it without any physical catastrophes, but I would not be so lucky. While in physical education class, I once again had a mishap. While playing volleyball just as I announced I had it, I proceeded to hit the ball. Only about two of my fingers were able to connect with the ball, it would bend one finger and the other little finger popped out of socket. As the bone protruded forward in the center of my little finger, I cried in pain. This time my middle school teacher would send me to the nurse, and my mother immediately took me to the emergency room. But after waiting for hours at the county hospital, the doctor finally merely walked up to me without giving me any medication and tugged, pulled, and wiggled my finger until it was back in place. I reeked out horrible screams while experiencing excruciating pain, as the doctor's treatment turned out to be even worst than the initial incident. The next day I mentioned to my PE teacher how painful it was and she was shocked, "You mean the doctor did not give you any medicine to deaden the finger. Oh my God, you all should have never gone to that County Hospital, you should have went to St. Elizabeth Hospital." In the years to come my finger would never be the same, as both fingers always look a bit swollen and crooked as they sometime pop while remaining rather stiff.

&ra; &ra; &ra; &ra; &ra; &ra; &ra; &ra; &ra; &ra; &ra; &ra; &ra; &ra; &ra; &ra; &ra; &ra;

As we approached the middle of the eight-grade I thought things started to get a little better, as a schoolmate named Ken started to follow me to my classes and carry my books. One day he made an abrupt turn toward the auditorium door, while grabbing my hand. As we stood in a dark entrance, he moved toward what would have been my first kiss. I recall I probably would have kissed him, but I just could not get over a strange but true vision in my mind. That was the fact that Ken had an awesome green plague, which lined the top of his front teeth.

I told one of my girlfriends what had happened, she would break out in a loud laugh and say, "You mean you passed up a chance to kiss that cute Ken because of his teeth. Girl you are crazy I bet I would have kissed him any way". I guess maybe I really did not like him that much, and maybe the teeth were just an excuse. One thing I did know and that was I wanted that moment to be perfect, or else I was not going to have a kiss. It would not be until high school before a moment like this was presented again.

But sometimes more of just merely trying to fit in took precedence over love. Trying to fit in was finding everything that you could wrong, with your clothes or your general physical appearance as well as your personality. I started to imagine that my ears were too large and spent a few weeks walking around with hands over my ears. Then one of my best friends decided she would become Bill Cosby's Fat Albert character, for the rest of the school year. So every time you would talk to her she would reply, "Hey, Hey, Hey, its Fat Albert. Nah, Nah, Nah, Going to have a good time". As she would walk around leaning slightly back a bit. As we would merely look at Mona in awe, and rarely talk to her because we knew she go into her Fat Albert routine every day. Those days were hard for everyone just as growing up and living day to day was a constant challenge for everyone. It was even harder for us to conceive, or comprehend that everyone else was going through the same identity dilemmas.

One of the more positive experiences I recall during eighth grade was vocational class with Mr. Holman, a nurturing and caring eight-grade instructor. Mr. Holman was a young tall handsome blonde man,

who was always very pleasant and greeted all his students with a huge
smile. He was a newlywed and would tell us stories about his innovative
and creative wife's endeavors to fix up the old house they just moved
into. He exclaimed, "The house looks great, I mean everything is color
coordinated. She painted everything from the walls to the toilet seat, as
well as the wallpaper. It is really nice." You could tell his excitement
and endless loving bliss when he spoke of this seemingly kindhearted
wife. This was the first instructor I felt free to voice my opinions, as he
would probe our psychic by asking us questions about our lives. After
the first few weeks of him making us feel comfortable enough to talk he
would ask. "I would like each one of you to tell me something about
yourself such as your favorite subject, what you want to be when you
grow up, and what you like to do for fun, for example, a hobby." As he
went down the first row of wooden tables aligned next to each other, it
was my turn to speak as he slowly approached the second row of tables.
One of my Spanish-Indian friends had recently showed me how to
connect, doublement gum papers together to make a replica of a bedded
doorway or even a belt. It was a fairly inexpensive hobby that only
required gathering my fellow students gum wrappers. The hobby also
proved to be rather abundant and fruitful as most of our classmates
endlessly chewed gum. As Mr. Holman made everyone feel so
comfortable, I would speak rather openly with little embarrassment for
the first time, "My favorite subject is math, I would like to help people
and maybe even become a doctor. My hobbies include writing and
making long strings of paper chains from doublement gum wrapper
paper." This teacher was such a professional as he replied very
responsively, "and you can connect these wrappers together". I would
continue to explain, "Yes we fold them and loop them together back and
forth into a zigzag shape." Mr. Holman smiled and would reply, How
interesting and amazing and what do you do with them." "We can use
them as belts or as a string of beads hanging from a doorway in the house
for privacy," as I confidently responded. "That is truly amazing and I
would like to see that if you would like to bring it in one day," he

exclaimed. The next day I demonstrated my hobby to the class and Mr. Holman was so receptive and full of encouragement.

All and all the rest of the year was good until the effects of chewing too much gum or drinking too much soda took its toll, as that same year I would develop a really bad infection. Helen would finally rush me to the emergency room, after I had been on my knees next to the bed for a couple of days suffering from severe abdomen pain. The doctor advised I had an infection around the appendix area but only gave me an antibiotic. He further advised if I did not get any better or if it reoccurred, he would have to remove my appendix. I lasted for a year without another episode, and after that year the same excruciating pain occurred once again.

That next year, 1974, the same excruciating pain occurred once again. After the surgery I stayed in the hospital about a week, and my mother stayed with me until I tried to send her home. But I was glad she stayed, as I was really afraid to be in the hospital alone. While I returned to school, I would not be able to walk up the steps for three months. During this time some of my classmates would always try to make me laugh as one guy attempted to imitate the Soul Train dancers. But as I finally returned to classes I learned one of my classmates was playing Russian roulette with his friends, and accidentally took his own life. After that most devastating event and I would look across the room at his empty seat, I figured maybe my problems were not as bad as I thought.

Immediately following the surgery, I went through a period of extreme withdrawal. I developed a condition of extreme fear and unrest, as there appeared to be some sort of an imbalance in my system after the surgery. My nutrition no doubt lacked horribly as I barely ate. Then anxiety started to set-in as every time I would go anywhere such as class, church, or any stressful situation, some most depressing and confused thoughts surfaced. As more and more negative feelings overtook every aspect of my life, there were times I would just pray so hard and long for God to help me day after day to overcome the depression. Another one of my Spanish classmates advised how her grandmother said someone can look at you, and put an 'evil eye' or a curse on you. She further advised you have to put an egg in a pan underneath your bed and if starts to cook, you have a curse. Once the egg fully cooks the curse is broken, and although I did not attempt this remedy I did have lot of people praying for me.

Finally one night while attending communion, our Pastor glanced over at me with a strange and concerned look. I didn't think anyone was aware of my distress. But when we passed by the pulpit to shake hands with the Pastor and deacons following the services, the Pastor just pulled my hand toward him. He then laid his hand on my head and prayed for me, "Lord in the name of Jesus. Satan release your hold on this child in the name of Jesus, I said in the mighty name of Jesus get out from this child". As he prayed I felt a peace come over me. I had not felt this extreme peace since my early childhood years. I knew in my heart that I had a miracle as all the strange feelings began to cease. For God healed me from those dysfunctional feelings and I never had an anxiety attack quite like that again.

Then oddly my love for writing started to emerge as I started to write short stories, poems, and even a few letters, which materialized into an even further healing. I guess it was my way of venting all of the pain as well as just trying to understand what life was really about for me. One of the first items I wrote was a letter to Stevie Wonder for some of his great musical works. As I never had a chance to mail the letter and still have the stamped envelope to Black Bull Press in New York. I did eventually use the letter as one of many short essay-writing assignments for my high school English class.

〰〰〰〰〰〰〰〰〰〰〰〰〰〰〰〰〰

Dear Mr. Wonder,

*I am writing you a letter from my deepest most inner thoughts. A letter that I feel only you, Mr. Wonder would understand. I don't know if you will ever receive this letter, but in my heart I will always feel you know how many of us cherish you just as I. I listen to your album over and over. It seems to become finer and finer every time I hear it. It touches a part of me that is very deep and real. It is beyond any of my thoughts and has touched a part of my soul that only your music touches. No one can reach the part of me that you do. Your music describes everything I feel inside and much more. A kind of music that tells life's true meaning and purpose. A kind of music that...that gives me an inspiration just burning inside. You give me an inspiration to want to go past and beyond my human capability. I wish to give everyone in the world the same happiness you give me. Music had no real meaning to me until you brought your song and words together. Song's that tell life's true meaning. A real truth in every song you sing. I could go on and on about your music Mr. Wonder, but I have to stop before I go beyond my own thoughts......but Stevie Wonder you are the music, the heart and soul of it. You are the greatest and thank you very much because now I can feel it all over....*

*Yours truly,*
*Signed Nanette*

## Chapter 4: Teenage Years 'Roller Coaster of Confusion'

Although my parents had their rules and regulations we had to follow, we felt after my father died, Helen, became too strict. But both my parents viewed a broader picture, which focused on their children's future success, and I must admit Daddy's spirit of education was deposited and still remains inside me. Since Daddy passed away when I was rather young, Helen often reiterated how my father desired that we all complete our education. I always kept a deep and passionate desire with much anticipation toward continuing my education. It would have been an historic event not only for me but also my father, as I delighted and looked forward to being the first generation of being able to graduate a four-year college. This deep desire and spirit of my father would no doubt somehow continue to dwell deep within me, even throughout my confusing and sometimes misled high school years and adult life.

When I entered high school I was still somewhat of a wallflower, as my brother had been in the hospital for months. He lost it to some bad drugs, as one day he returned home from school talking out of his mind. He played one of his records over and over before he finally lost it all together, I will never forget the horrifying experience as my Uncle had to not only run after and tackle my brother but restrain him with his hand cuffs. It was so sad to see my brother restrained and talking out of his head. It was very traumatic for the entire family. Just thinking about it makes the tears flow again. We went to see him often and one day I thought my mother was about to loose it, as she had a fit and crying rage as she left my brother's jacket in the hospital lobby.

He would eventually return to school and marry one of his high school classmates, Ella. They were fine for about a year as they took my sister from the college game room to driving lessons or just visiting friends.

☹ ❦ ❦ ❦ ❦ ❦ ❦ ☹

I eventually made friends with one classmate in my homeroom. She liked to joke around and we got along real well as we talked about boys mostly. Felicia was in love with Gary and talked about how much they were in love most of the time. One day after school Felicia had gone over his house and no one was home. She said Gary advised he loved her unlike he loved anyone else, and of course one thing led to another. Not long afterwards, Felicia started to act strange and began gaining weight. When we would go to our lockers she would yell at people around her to move, and even started to lash out by striking one of our classmates. My locker was right next to Felicia's, and just like everyone else we began to wonder what was wrong with her.

One Saturday Felicia came by the house. My niece was running through the house, which at the time was not a strange occurrence, and Felicia said, "You're getting ready to run track pretty soon, just keep practicing". We laughed and then she finally told me she was pregnant, but lost the baby. That was the last real conversation we had with each other as best friends. Not long after Felicia lost the first baby, she was pregnant again. She left school for good to attend the high school for expectant mothers. Needless to say my mother was not very open, as we were not allowed to go anywhere unless we had proper supervision. It would not be until years later that I would eventually understand my mother's reasoning, as I just thought she was being too old fashioned and strict with us.

After Felicia left I became friends with a couple of girl's from New York, Shiara and her sister, Monica, who were originally born in Columbia. I thought they were very mature for their ages, and I later found they were older than we thought. Shiara wanted to share lockers with me because she said she did not have a lock. Although I eventually thought the only reason why she became my friend was to get closer to Murray, who was in my homeroom. As I would eventually introduce them, and she began to very indiscreetly appear everywhere Murray was. Once we were eating lunch and although we had assigned seating with our homeroom class, Shiara would come over and sit next to us. If Murray was interested in anyone else, they did not have a chance because Shiara was always right there. She would laugh at anything he said and talked about him day and night. "Oh this guy is so funny. Ha...Ha... Did you hear what he said Nanette. Ha...Ha...Ha....". Shiara was a couple of years older than I was and once she decided on Murray I believe she must have thrown away the key. In the meantime, I started to become interested in Damion, another guy in our homeroom. After we continued to talk for a few weeks, I knew he would eventually want to kiss me so I asked Monica and Shiara what to do. Monica explained, "Just open your mouth and push out your tongue", as I would respond how gross, we started to giggle. As Ernest, a Spanish guy would pass down the hallway looking and smiling at us said, "I know y'all talking bout me, Huh, I know", as he rubs his chin smiling. Although I did think he was kind of cute too. Generally speaking every other boy was kind of cute during these teenage years.

But I was drawn to Damion as he had a rugged, handsome look with muscles and he bounced slightly as he walked on his toes. Damion played football and I fell madly in love with Damion after our first kiss in the first floor stairwell. As he started to kiss me very tenderly and softly, I told him it was my first kiss and he smiled. Then he continued to kiss me and as he kissed my neck, I just melted. Afterwards he walked me to the bus stop and we did not want to leave each other. All I could think about was Damion for the entire trip home, as well as that night.

Finally Damion asked for my phone number and I responded, "I have to ask my mother first, as she does not really allow me to date yet." That evening when I asked her I knew what her answer would be. Felicia had just recently left school because of her pregnancy so Helen's response was as I had imagined, "You are too young to even be thinking about boys". Then I responded, "We are only going to talk Helen and he's nice, and you can talk to him". But Helen was very stern and replied, "I said no, so stop asking me about that girl and that's final. You are too young, you're only fifteen years old. You do not have any business trying to date boys." Damion called that same night, and I advised him I could not talk. He even offered to talk to Helen. I tried to hand my mother the phone and said, "He wants to talk to you." All he could hear was Helen saying in the background was, "No, I said no, you cannot receive phone calls from any boys. Now you had better hang up pretty quick".

I was devastated to say the least, and that very next day I talked to Monica. I told her all about it and she fired up. She said, " it will make you feel better because our parents don't understand us." Monica's boyfriend was in New York and she wanted to be with him, but her parents would not allow that. Monica ran away several times in New York and she said she was going to run away again and go back to New York. "Once Hulio sends for me girl, I am gone. I mean I am out of here, bye-bye", as she gets high and starts laughing.

After that I seriously thought about running away. I loved to write short stories so that week I started to write about a girl who ran away. She lived on the street, ate out of garbage cans, and woke up on park benches. But she loved her boyfriend and every chance she found she was hugging and kissing him. I guess writing was good therapy as it became an outlet for venting my painful feeling. A few weeks later my sister told me Damion was dating one of the cheerleaders, Sharon. I knew it could not be true, as Damion had deep feelings for me. Then she advised how she saw Sharon kissing him in the hallway. I could not believe it until one night while my brother had taken us to a football game, and as Damion ran out on the field they grabbed hands. In an effort to forget about Damion and this most messed up situation, I started looking at other guys. I thought maybe I could give Ernest a chance. He appeared to have some interest in me, but then I saw him walking down the hallway holding hands with someone else. I could not make this situation right, and I was so alone and depressed.

Feeling bad about everything with Damion and my mother's rules and regulations, I reached a turning point. As I did not realize it was her way of trying to protect me. Then I made a conscious decision to do something I was taught not to my whole life. I wanted to rebel against my mother. So although I knew it was wrong, I attempted to smoke. One day as Monica was smoking in the girls' room, I started to smoke as well. This was the turning point, and my life started to take the wrong turn. When we finished smoking she helped me put on this deep shade of purple lipstick. I loved it although I felt embarrassed as I walked down the hallway laughing. As we walked and laughed it seemed to make me feel better if only for that moment.

That Saturday my older brother, Charles, had his wife's old 1968 thunderbird and took me over Shiara and Monica's house. Although Monica was glad to see me, Shiara was rather withdrawn. As Monica pulled me in her room and started talking Shiara slowly followed. Her parents looked at me strange and I guess that was because they thought I might be trouble. Little did they know their daughters taught me everything I knew.

ᎠᎠᎠᎠᎠᎠᎠᎠᎠᎠᎠᎠᎠᎠ

Another friend Sara, whom I met during our high school French class, had waist length extremely straight black hair. Although she was fair-skinned she often spoke of how her hair was just like Indian grandmother, and conveyed it would not curl at all. She talked about her adult boyfriend everyday during class and although I talked and tried to maintain these friendships, it would only make me fell even more out of place as I started to experience problems in school. Feeling out of place and unable to identify very well with my peers, simply because I was not allowed to socialize outside of school, gave rise to more incidents as my teenage dilemmas appeared so enormous and vast at the time.

The next major bazaar incident occurred during a school bazaar while I sat across the room from some students. One student appeared to have said something, he looked over and whispered back and they started to laugh. Afterwards I stood up, yelled at them, and stormed out of the room as I felt all the built up frustration emerge. In the next few weeks to come, I began feeling even more inadequate. As we could not often times afford new clothes I had to wear hand me downs, and because I didn't dress as good as some of the other kids I exhibited even more feelings of insecurity.

As these insecurities finally peaked during physical education class as I was sitting in a corner alone in deep thought, and the teacher yelled, "Get up and go pick up the archery arrows." I drug myself up very slowly and walked listlessly. The teacher, Ms. Moss was furious, she thought I was trying to be disobedient. "I am going to call your mother right now young lady", she resounded. I pleaded with her not to call, but as it turned out Helen immediately came to the school. Our family friend Mrs. Moore drove her there, and they both said, "How can you call a parent about a child not picking up an arrow fast enough, right in the middle of your class period. What is the real meaning of this? Did she do something else or has she ever been a problem before. Well this is outrageous and I will be talking to the principal about this". Helen stormed out of the office and from that day on I always received low grades in her class, even though I studied for the test.

After I keep receiving low grades Helen decided to transfer me to Jack Yates High School, only to embark upon more extraordinary experiences.

ꙅ ꙅ ꙅ ꙅ ꙅ ꙅ ꙅ ꙅ ꙅ ꙅ ꙅ ꙅ ꙅ ꙅ ꙅ ꙅ

As I transferred from Austin Senior High, I had taken a Journalism course and was well versed in the subject matter. So, when I signed up for Journalism at Yates I was able to answer all the questions in class and Ms. Jones was impressed as she asked, "Can anyone tell me the 'four W's and the 'H' in journalism?" I responded immediately without hesitation with, "Who, what, when, where, and how". From there I was asked to write for the paper and would join the yearbook staff as well. Some of my work in the newspaper included poems as well as articles. The writing seemed to sometimes help ease my distressed feelings. Our student teacher could not believe I wrote the poem entitled 'Can It Be', and he literally challenged me for a few minutes on the issue. I could not figure out why as I thought he must have felt it was some great literary work, but it would no doubt inspire me to continue to write even more poems.

*Can It Be?*
*Can It Be that life is only a game we play,*
*Can it be that we are all living in Hell, and Heaven is our death.*
*Can it be that our lives are very short, and hard to live and yet pleasant.*
*Can it be we can live our lives without hurting another? Can it be?*
*Can it be that living is a dream, and love is only our hearts sorrow?*
*Can it be that marriage is something man created to keep a love from leaving?*
*Can it be?*

℞ ℞ ℞ ℞ ℞ ℞ ℞ ℞ ℞ ℞ ℞ ℞ ℞ ℞ ℞ ℞ ℞ ℞ ℞

*'My Philosophy of Life'*
*I feel love is life and love is happiness. Life is precious and needs not to be wasted or abused in any way. You should live life for all it's worth. I love life and feel every moment should be lived with love. Loving one another and caring one for another. The sharing of heartache and the sharing of pain. The feeling of love for someone special. The feeling of being loved by someone special. Life is filled with love and you can make it happen. We can make life beautiful for ourselves, and the world around.*

℞ ℞ ℞ ℞ ℞ ℞ ℞ ℞ ℞ ℞ ℞ ℞

As the editor of the editorial section of our paper, I wrote on various issues of concern and proofread other writer's editorials. The article below was written for our high school paper entitled, The Lion's Tale for the March 2, 1977 issue. This editorial was no doubt ahead of its time, because drug prevention was virtually unheard of. But it appears someone was paying attention to what we were crying out for, as drug prevention for young people has developed a great deal since the 70's. Maybe my little voice played a role in today's drug prevention, as it has extended throughout the school system and society including the using major media such as television as vehicles. Little did anyone know the following editorial, would be my own personal cry for help.

"Drugs Seen As A Major Problem Today"
By Nanette Broussard
"Drugs are a very large problem in schools today. High School students who cannot cope with reality; often turn to drugs to ease their tensions. Drugs are widespread in high schools, junior high schools, and even in elementary schools. Millions of students everyday are being introduced to drugs as a "way out...a way to rid themselves of their problems and begin a better life...a better way of life that often ends in terrible tragedies. Students are becoming more and more obsessed with drugs. Every day this murderer called drugs strikes out at the often ill-fated youthful offenders. No one knows who the next victim will be.
Who knows how we can stop this killer?
What can we do to help one that is hooked on drugs?
We cannot solve or answer all these questions, but we must try.
I personally feel that more material and coverage should be provided to students. I feel if more students knew what problem drugs can cause them, there would be less usage. Students should be able to obtain more knowledge on the principle effects of these monsters called drugs."

ᄭ ᄭ ᄭ ᄭ ᄭ ᄭ ᄭ ᄭ ᄭ ᄭ ᄭ ᄭ ᄭ ᄭ ᄭ ᄭ ᄭ

This article on drugs was most ironic as I watched our principal chase the drug dealers off the campus, and the schools only blatantly open teenage addict staggers down the hallway only to be expelled once again. I will never forget the sad sight, as he was one of the best-dressed teenagers in the school, while constantly stoned out of his mind nearly all the time. Needless to say he was not seen at the graduation ceremonies.

The next few editorials included articles and hot topics from the importance of homeroom attendance to the need for better restroom sanitary conditions. I also wrote a story on a field trip in Oceanography class to Galveston. We took the ferry to Bolivar Peninsula, and I recall standing near the bow of the ship and watching the water very closely. As I began to lean over the railing, it was as though my mind and body was so relaxed and free. Just then, a guy in class walked up and covered his whole body over me. I believe my teacher saw me at the rail, and advised him to watch me because he followed the whole time we were on the boat. Later, while we were on the beach my sandal broke rendering me barefoot. I was so embarrassed. As I walked with my sandals in my hands, it was as though I was never as good as everyone else. It just magnified my current situation, the feelings of being poor in every since of the word. My teacher offered to take me home, and I felt extreme relieve only for a moment but the bad feelings soon returned. As she got closer to my house, I would ask her drop me off on the corner. I did not want anyone to see where I lived since this type of house was termed a shotgun house, because it was as straight as the barrel of a shotgun. Needless to say I was rather embarrassed, because one could go from the front to the back of the house and would have walked through every room. As a teenager this house somehow made me feel so ashamed, as the recently painted pastel green paint was already starting to peel. As she slowed down, nearing my street I advised, "I can get out here". She insisted on dropping me off at my house, and proceeded to turn. Once we arrived at my house, she said, "I think you have a very nice house". This lady was not only a very good teacher but also a very caring individual, who no doubt could read every negative thought on my mind and handled this situation most tactfully. I thank God for teachers like

Ms. Jesuite, because if it had been handled otherwise, it could have been even more devastating. By Ms. Jesuite reaching out in this matter helped to ease some of my negative feelings, and although I would go on to make some mistakes I would also make many good choices as well because of some most positive role models.

But although I did continue to get involved with more negative influences, I somehow kept my ultimate educational goal. I felt more withdrawn from the mainstream even though I began to acquire much attention. I even recall one of the members of our church always saying to my mother, that's the pretty one. Even when I went to pick up my high school graduation pictures the photographer renounced, "I know you are Miss Yates". As I would just shyly smile and respond no. I never really thought of myself as one of the pretty girls, but I guess subconsciously I enjoyed the attention. The continued attention would not help curtail the many unwarranted decisions I made in my life, but rather possibly add to them.

As our yearbook budget had been in the red for a couple of years, we tried to raise funds. We soliciting ads for our school paper, but this wonderful attempt merely ended up as a failed attempt to gain funds for our 1978 yearbook. Although we had to forfeit our class yearbook printing that year due to a deficit school budget, the next year's graduating class did include our graduating class. I guess all was not lost as they combined the graduating class of 1978 with the graduating class of 1979 publication.

After not being able to sell the newspaper, we eventually decided to give the plain white folded or stapled sheets away. We further changed the name of our newspaper to the 'Lion's Roar', in an effort to attract more student readers. It appeared to help as more people started to read the paper, seeing that I started to receive a few comments on my articles. Not long after my rein of articles, I was voted the yearbook sweetheart. As I did not have a boyfriend at the time, I asked a classmate to escort me. All the sweethearts had to parade onto the field during half time at the homecoming football game. I had on a white suit, my corsage, and my banner draped across entitled 'Yearbook Sweetheart

1978', which is now one of my keepsakes from the past. My escort, Chris, had a nice gray suit and really big hair as we looked great and took lots of pictures. His girlfriend seemed to be fine with the situation, but he eventually left me sitting on the bleacher alone. His girlfriend called him away to sit with her during the rest of the game. I understood as he excused himself politely, and I would cherish being in the homecoming event forever.

While working on the newspaper staff I met Princes. She was a classmate who was on the newspaper and yearbook staff with me. Princes loved to wear lots of make up, which was something my mother was not very fund of. She further lived with her boyfriend after running away from her home. This was no doubt my first brush on the wild side of life that I would never forget and have many regrets.

I remember one day Princes and I had planned to go to the movies on Saturday, but when she drove up with her boyfriend my mother went ballistic. Princes wore heavy make up and had very thick eyelashes with liner, eye shadow, bright lipstick, and skimpy clothes. My mother would ask me where did I meet that woman, and when I advised her she was a high school student she did not believe it. "You are telling me that woman is in high school, she looks like a streetwalker. Where did you meet up with her at?" "I told you Helen, she goes to school with me, she is only seventeen." "Huh seventeen, I know better than that. That is an old hard knot that's been on the road a long time, and furthermore you are not going any where with her and that's final. Now go tell her you cannot go." Well as I walked slowly toward her car she asked, "What's the problem"? "I can't go, my mother said I can't go to the movies with you guys". Princes advised, "What, why can't you go with us. Why, just let me talk to her", as she gets out of car and walks back toward the house. "We just going to the movies, why you won't let her go." Helen advised, "Look I said Nanette is not going to the movies with you all." "But why you won't let her go", as Princes continued to push the issue. Helen replied very forcefully, "Because I said so, that's why. And Nanette you need to hurry up and come in this house." Princes gave Helen a look and just shook her head as we walked back toward the car. "I can't believe your mother, man what's wrong with her, why is she strict. Girl please, now are you going or not?" I told Princes that maybe we would go another time. As they drove off, Helen continued to tell me to stay away from her. My mother was absolutely right in her analysis of the situation, but I continued to rebel. I was very impressionable and continued to look in the wrong places for friendship. As I yearned to be recognized as a maturing young lady capable of making my own decisions, and just wanted to go out sometimes and also a possible occasional date. All the while not quite understanding my mother's views or concerns, as she did not sometimes fully explain 'the why not' very clearly. I never dreamed she was trying to avoid what was about to unfold, while I continued to choose most inappropriate acquaintances. I often times wish my mother would have let me date, and just told me how to take care of myself. Maybe there is a possibility that if she had known whom I was dating, I would not have been taken advantage of. Furthermore, I wished someone had taught how to fight back. Such as self-defense or told how to kick a would-be sex offender in the balls. It is no doubt very clear to me that you cannot stop your children from growing up, but it is vital to know who they are with and teach them how to take of themselves. As I often wonder if it would have helped me.

But I continued to mistakenly turn my life in the wrong direction while continuing to write about my inner most thoughts and frustrations.


✠ ✠ ✠ ✠ ✠ ✠ ✠ ✠ ✠ ✠ ✠ ✠ ✠ ✠ ✠ ✠ ✠ ✠ ✠ ✠ ✠ ✠

*What is Freedom?*
*Have you ever stopped and asked yourself what is Freedom?*
*Just wondered what the word was all about.*
*Is it a word to justify free, maybe just a mere fantasy?*
*A figment of our blind imaginations that only last*
*as long as we let it.*
*Upon our own heart, soul, body,*
*and mind sit the word to create either peace or chaos.*
*No, this word is not just mere letters*
*but rather our own vulnerable understanding of Freedom.*
*Not to do what we want, and never lasting forever.*
*Freedom, What is Freedom?*

✠ ✠ ✠ ✠ ✠ ✠ ✠ ✠ ✠ ✠ ✠ ✠ ✠ ✠ ✠ ✠ ✠ ✠ ✠ ✠ ✠

That night after the movie controversy, Princes called and Helen advised me not to have anything to do with her and to hurry up and get off the phone. Not long after that travesty occurred in my life, the saga would continue to plague my already confused life. As I would eventually realize, my mother really did sometimes know best.

One afternoon as we were waiting for the bus as usual, Princes decided to wave down a passing car for a ride. It was a nice brand new royal blue Chevrolet ninety-eight with a white top and sunroof. He was nice looking and well-dressed gentleman as Princes tried so hard to get me to get in that car. "Come on Nanette, he's going to give us a ride come here." As I reluctantly walked over to the car he said, "Hi, I'm Wesley, but everyone calls me West. Hey, what's your name". "Nanette", I said very softly. "You want a ride, I mean I'll take you wherever y'all wanna go, come on." " No, I don't think so", I responded. Princes repeatedly saying as she gets in the car, "Come on girl, I'll ride with you". Princes then gets into the car and stretches her arms across the back relaxing, "Come on girl". As I slowly got in the front seat West said, "Where you going." " I live down this street just turn here", as I did want him to know exactly where I lived. Helen would have had a fit if she saw me riding with a stranger. Right before I got out of the car he asked, "Well Nanette, Can I call you sometime?" " I then answered, "No, I don't think so, you can drop me off right here at the corner". "Okay, well you can call me anytime", as West wrote his phone number down and smiled.

I remember falling for him as I started to call him daily, and I eventually invited him to my high school sweetheart ball. As the yearbook sweetheart, I had to walk up on the stage and curtsy to our high school queen and her court. That night I had my sister drop me off, and Helen did not know about West.

I recall when West showed up everyone thought he was my older brother, as West was in his mid-twenties. I heard a couple of comments like, "Who is that? He's a little young for her Daddy, so it must be her brother. But he is really cute, ooh wee."

As I stood there with West with my dress being a slight bit too long, but just having a handsome guy on my arm made me fell beautiful anyway. As soon as the program was over, West asked to take me home. One of my girlfriends was with me that night and advised she would ride with us. We were all just riding around, as he started to get us a high. West was kissing me every chance he could, as he was a great kisser I thought.

Then as we arrived at Linda's place she tried to get me out of the car, as we dropped her off first. "Come on Nanette, you come on in and we'll take you home later", Linda insisted. But I felt like West could drop me off so I said, "no I'll be okay, West will take me home."

As we drove off to what I thought would be my house, he made what I thought was a wrong turn. "Oh, I live down that way remember". "Well we are going to take a little ride first". He frightened me with his demeanor, and I started to get very nervous. As he continued to drive farther and farther away, I thought I may never see anyone alive again and started to plead with him. "But I cannot go anywhere else with you, I am already late and I need to go home or my mother will have a fit. Please just take me home West." He would not respond and simply ignored my pleads and by the time he did reply, I was in total fear.

Finally once he arrived at his apartment he said, "We're only going to be a little while, I want to show you where I live. Now get out of the car".

I did not want to get out of the car but as we drove into his complex he said, "come on up just a little while. I just want to show you my place that's all. Now we have drove all this way and you might as well get out of the car, okay", as he smiles and kisses me softly. I proceeded to slowly get out of the car as he pulled and held my arm as we entered the apartment he said, "Here is my living room. This is the kitchen, over here is the bathroom, which I am sure you need right about now. Am I right", as he smiles and kisses me. "Yea, I can use that right about now", as I went into the rest room. When I came out I looked and called out his name, "West". "I'm in here", he called. I walked around the corner to see him undressed to his shorts, and as I turned to walk away he grabbed me. He said, "Come here and tried to kiss me again". As I stopped the kiss and said, "Listen West I need to go. I can't. Please let me go home. Please I'll come back and see you another day. I'm just tired tonight". West persisted and would not let me go, as I must have stood against the wall trying to talk him out of it for what seemed to be a lifetime. He would not let me go and as he pulled me down, which was not difficult as I was already weak and feeling faint from the pleading and the minuscule but extended struggle. All I could remember is fighting to keep my clothes on, as I continually asked him to stop and did not have enough strength to stop him. Then I will never forget the pain I felt during the whole act. That night when he dropped me off he would leave me at the corner, and as I walked in the door Helen had a fit. She was yelling where have you been as I just replied with my girlfriend. For a moment I thought she would hit me, but eventually she settled down and I guess she sensed something was not right about me that night. But I knew I could not tell anyone especially my mother, as I felt it was all my fault.

He telephoned me continuously for weeks following the incident. As my mother called me to the phone, he would get some lady to call for him. He said on one occasion, "I need to see you. I bought you a ring. Please, when can I see you."? I would always reply, I don't know but I have to go. I guess the ring was an effort to ease his guilty conscious, but after I did not want to see him he eventually stopped calling. I just merely thought this horrible memory would fade from my very soul, and I felt it was my fault for even talking to an older man. He was about twenty-five years old and I did kiss him, but I was not even thinking of becoming intimate with anyone yet. I don't know if I would have ever been with West if he hadn't raped me. All I knew was that he took something from me that I was not yet willing or ready to give. I guess this was one of the major negative incidents in my life that would ultimately affect and even dictate how I dealt with all my future relationships. My only regret is that I wished I had told an adult, not necessarily for revenge, but to release myself from the horrible haunting silent pain. Now I realize after all these years of wasted and bad relationships that I should have sought out some professional help. From that day on I was disconcerted and degraded love making as merely an act, rather than the beautiful and wondrous ultimate display of love I thought it should be.

I recall the next day on the bus, Linda looked at me and tears just started to run down my face. She shook her head and said, "I knew that twenty-five year old man was not going to take you straight home. That's why I tried to get you to get out of that car girl. I tried to get you out of that car girl." Linda saw all the pain I was feeling in my face, as I sat and looked her. After graduation I saw Linda a few times and eventually she confided in me how she had been raped as well. How naive was I to think I could trust a man that I really knew nothing about. The one thing my mother tried so hard to protect me from would inevitably end up happening once again.

For months to come I would avoid the bus stop where I met West as well as Princes, sometimes I would walk further down to another stop or often times I would just walk home. I preferred not to see either one of them.

Eventually I acquired a part time job at the local University, and I was really excited. My mother was not very happy about it as she exclaimed, "Why do you girls always want to work. You do not need to be working." I guess my mother was just overprotective and rightfully so. Although I knew most of my life I wanted to attend college, there was another side of me, which subconsciously searched for that homemaker life. Only because it was the way I was raised, as my mother was a homemaker, and did not work until my father fell ill with heart trouble. But it was not necessarily all I wanted, I longed also for the college life and felt so excited about the idea of one day attending college. I further reveled in the idea that I could work and make my own money, as well as relished in the eventual opportunity to be independent.

After being elated upon receiving my first paycheck, I decided to give it to my mother. But she did not have any intention of taking any money from me, and would only say, "you keep it. It's your money, and you should spend it on yourself". I went directly downtown and purchased some records. I bought Bootsie Collins, George Clinton, Peter Frampton, and Stevie Wonder's hit 2 record album set with a 21 page lyric book, 'Songs In The Key of Life'. And I also loved to listen to the little something extra record called 'Saturn'. I would listen to that record over and over as it described me and how I desired to leave all the past behind, and just go away. I would later on purchase a couple of outfits with the subsequent paychecks. Finally after feeling a sense of pride for once in a long time, I started feeling pretty good about me. I later returned to purchase more brand new clothes, no more hand me downs for me. I was making money now and loving every minute of it. Although I was only able to put clothes in lay-a-way, I felt like I was living life for the first time. After only receiving a few paychecks, the director of this government funded program advised my assignment would be ending soon. I can remember feeling so alone and insecure again. Then as I stood waiting for the bus that afternoon, a stranger stopped and offered me a ride. He was rather persistent and for some unknown reason at the time, I finally said yes. I was probably just feeling sad and vulnerable after loosing my job, because I knew better than to do that again.

After I got into the car, I knew it was not what I should have done and I immediately began to silently pray. I knew this man was no good as I felt his eyes all over me, and did want history to repeat itself. As I told him where to turn, he looked at me and reluctantly turned the corner. Then finally I advised, "can you let me off here". He said, "I can take you home. Why don't you let me drop you off at your door". "No", I insisted, "just let me off right here". As he finally slowed down, God must have heard my prayers as I walked quickly down the street. I looked around, as it seemed the longest block I ever walked.

Sometimes I felt my impulsive and unexplained actions were due to the date rape. And although I did have good parents, they could not take away my pain. It was as though I relived the childhood molestation all over again, but this time it resurfaced never to be forgotten again. It would haunt me and try to dictate the rest of my unsettling life. Once I continued to concentrate on the negative aspects of my life, the insecurity literally took over my entire being. I felt I could never measure up or compete with anyone. Only a select few in which I ended up befriending. Most of my friends did drugs or drank heavily and partied, and I felt not only accepted but it also helped me forget the pain. As I continued to write my poems, I now know subconsciously I was crying out. Not realizing it at the time there was a war going on deep down within my soul, but one thing I did know and that was I did not want to live my life without achieving my most cherished dreams and I had to continue to fight for it. As I proclaimed in the next two poems.

δδδδδδδδδδδδδδδδδδδδδδδδδδδδδδδδδδδδδδδ

### 'Drugs Wont' Conquer'

Drugs wont' conquer, though some have said so
Powerful and devastating you are, not so.
Some think you will overthrow us and consume us all,
But don't trip because you wont' kill me.
You are like a plague that infests our youth.
A high above all others is what they say,
And some of our best men you did take
Rest in their bones, and soul's delivery.
You enslave men women, whether they are black or white
With your sickness, corruptness, and betrayal coincide.
But we will burst with pride and enthusiasm, for we have won.
There will be no eternal rest, from your plague
And you will rein no more, Drugs You Will Die!!!


.: .: .: .: .: .: .: .: .: .: .: .: .:


### 'You May Think'

You may think that all life is fun and games,
You may think.
Live and let live,
You may think.
Just have fun for tomorrow is another day of fun,
You may think.
For you may think that drinking and getting a high is great,
But I bet you have never stopped to think of what you may think in the future.
Maybe you will think confused, poor, or maybe even crazy,
You may think.
For we all may think now because in the future you may cannot.


⋇ ⋇ ⋇ ⋇ ⋇ ⋇ ⋇ ⋇ ⋇ ⋇ ⋇ ⋇ ⋇ ⋇ ⋇ ⋇

Not long after the rape, the Pastor's son started to come by more often as we lived right across the street from the church. Finally, one night while we talked on the phone he advised, "Let me speak to your mother". I was like what, "No matter what you ask her, she will say no". "Well just let me talk to her", he said as I reluctantly gave my mother the phone. I could not believe Helen agreed to let me go out with a boy. I believe the only reason my mother agreed to let me date Horace was without a doubt, because he was the Pastor's son. But whatever her reasoning was, I was flabbergasted as I was seventeen years old almost eighteen and about to go on my very first official date.

Not long after we started to date during my senior year of high school, we started talking about my prom. I advised Horace I would be graduating early and would not be attending my prom. He advised I could still go to my prom and he would like to take me, but I refused. "I am not coming back to this school once I graduate." Horace tried to talk me into it as he said, "You got to go to your prom. I mean it's a once in a lifetime thing, and something you can look back at when you get old and treasure." As he continued to talk, it was as though I was in another world. Subconsciously still in shock and virtually lost trying to make sense of the life after losing my virginity before I wanted. I could not let go of the pain and all I wanted to do was to try to get away from everything. Nothing appeared to be happening like I wished it too, as deep down I was not really in control of my life. Nor did I have any clue of how to control my life, so I decided to just handle all the pain as best I could. As I advised Horace I did not want to attend my prom.

The following is a portion of one of the last pieces I wrote before graduation as I tried to make some sense of my life, while unknowingly inspiring myself to continue my hopes and dreams. As these feelings of hope continued to surface but would sometimes end up crushed by the never-ending pain inside.

*'A Letter to the Seniors'*

*'The graduating senior is no doubt a very fragile human being. He/She can be persuaded or even confused as life's transition to adulthood occurs most abruptly. The way in which they may lead their lives depends primarily on their surroundings. Their perception of life will affect the world and this perception stems from the surrounding environment. Character and moral standards they maintain are vital to America's well-being.............As I reminisce on this country's past history I feel sorrowful, and yet very determined. Determined to fulfill the dream of freedom of religion as well as education.*
*A dream of our forefathers to make a great land and this is a great land for all men and women. A dream burning deep inside their hearts and within their souls. A dream that only can be fulfilled by you, the graduating senior............*

&❖❖❖❖❖❖❖❖❖❖&

On our first date Horace and I went to the drive in movies, and I let him kiss me. Then he tried to touch me even further, and due to my recent abuse incident I did not stop him. But he stopped himself as he kept saying, "I cannot believe you are so sweet and Sister Broussard's' daughter". He was in shock just as much as I was as I did not know how to deal with this recent turn of events of being raped and I still told no one. He knew something was different about me, as he sometimes would just look at me. Our next few dates would be much the same as we attending various concerts a well, and every time we saw each other in church he would say how his grandmother said he should marry me. But I was too messed up to marry at that time. I was like a mindless and confused zombie, a wounded animal as I sought comfort any way I could. Never realizing it would only make the pain even worst. It was as though I had loss all my inner most feelings, and yet I knew I wanted and needed to love someone and to be loved. As my good judgment about love had been distorted, and all emotional control had been taken away from me. My feelings were useless because I felt no one cared about my feelings, and whom it was did not quite seem as important. I felt the only way to be loved was to let the man have his way.

I guess the date that stands out the most with Horace was our George Clinton concert. I had such fun, dressed up in my off white slacks and cream-colored sheer blouse. Although we were at the very top level of the auditorium, I still got up and danced. Horace just looked on as I shook very conservatively. Afterwards, he said he could not believe I got up and danced. After the concert he would once again bring up marrying me but being so emotionally disconnected, I never really gave him a straight answer. But finally after we drove around for a while that night in circles he advised me, "I decided to join the Navy". "Navy, but why" I replied. "Well I get to travel, and be on my own for awhile". After he dropped this revelation on me he would finally get a response out of his marriage proposal, "I cannot believe you. What do you want me to do? Well if you want me to wait, I think we should at least get engaged". So that weekend, we bought a beautiful little diamond ring solitaire that I still cherish to this day. That was as close to a real marriage I ever got, as I believe he really loved me in a very special way. Before he left we would talk daily and stayed on the phone for hours as he would sometimes read the Bible to me as if he were reading a wonderful storybook. I sometimes could not fully understand the old English of the Bible, but Horace interpreted it well and the words flowed smoothly and very plainly. And after reading he would eventually get real quiet as he talked himself to sleep, I would sometimes have to raise my voice to try and wake him to hang up the phone. "Horace wake up, wake up and hang the up. Horace", as I sometimes would go on for what seemed like hours. Being a slight bit too meticulous I did not want to hang up and leave him sleep on the phone, but once after growing rather frustrated I had to just hang up.

I felt quite comfortable with Horace. I loved being with him because he gave me a sense of safety, that I had not felt since my father passed. Horace sent the payments for the ring faithfully, but we eventually drifted apart and broke off the engagement after his discharge. I guess my life was to complicated as I had started to party rather regular.

As I wrote him often and sent tons of pictures and he wrote me as well, but it was not enough to keep us together. I was too busy partying too think about marrying, and I enjoyed making my own money as I loved independence. I also enjoyed attending college.

℗ ⁓⁓ ⁓⁓ ⁓⁓ ⁓⁓ ⁓⁓ ⁓⁓ ⁓⁓ ⁓⁓ ⁓⁓ ⁓⁓ ⁓⁓ ⁓⁓ ⁓⁓ ⁓⁓ ⁓⁓ ⁓⁓ ⁓⁓ ⁓⁓

I found my second job upon graduating early from high school at a McDonalds, as my mother would still exclaim, "I can't understand why you girls want to work". I believe Helen would have preferred we stay home with her all day. But I loved working and making my own money, and learning about life. While the job would only last about three weeks I would meet some truly opinionated young people who gave me plenty of unwarranted insight. One day after work a couple of my coworkers sat at the bus stop with me, and started a conversation about guys. Being the young most impressionable seventeen year old that I was, I listened most subjectively. "I cannot sleep with a man the first night I meet him, I mean I need to know him at least three weeks", one of the my coworkers said boldly as she lit her cigarette. I would not respond as I thought to myself, three weeks is not a whole lot of time. Although I am sure there was some logic to her reasoning, I could not help but note that love was not a part of the relationship. As I learned from most of the young people I knew that being in love with someone was not a major concern or prerequisite in having a relationship.

After about three weeks of working at McDonalds, Felicia whom I continued to keep in contact with after high school advised her brother, Leonard, who worked at a mortgage company downtown could probably get me on. As I used his name as a reference, and was so nervous as I walked into the VP's office for my first formal interview. It must have went very well, as they called me back immediately and I worked there for almost year before leaving. This job gave me good experience and allowed career enrichment and growth. It gave me enough stability to take a driving course at the local community college, and enabled me to purchase my first car. Although it would be years later after I purchased the car, before I actually learned how to drive.

Chapter 5: Adult Life 'Lost and Turned Out'

      After I turned eighteen years old, I felt compelled to do pretty much like I wanted as a lost young and confused adult. But I did have limits on what I did because of how Helen raised us, even after Daddy died. Basically I tried to keep Gods laws in my heart and the love of God was resident in my soul. I still often prayed between all the heartbreak as I was from one bad relationship after another.

      After Horace and I broke off the engagement as we had grown apart because the long distance of the relationship, I started to date another guy I went to high school with. Brian appeared to be a nice guy also as well. He had been trying to get hired on with the Postal Service and always told me how he would be hired and he did. Brian eventually acquired a very nice apartment, which was a major step up from the ward. But he had a Doberman that I could not get used to, but I tried to adjust. One night after I had stayed over, I took my pure tri-gold watch off in his bathroom. Not realizing it was missing until the next day, I asked Brian for my watch but to my surprise Brian said he did not see any watch. I figured he probably either gave it away or one of his other girlfriends probably came across it by accident. However, after this happened I never saw Brian again as I decided to file a police report.

      Later that same year I quit the mortgage company and began working at another company. As the neighborhood continued to become less safe and there was always something happening, my mother would pray to one day be able to move. Once I turned twenty-one, Helen, Sophia, and I moved from the ward into a subdivision on the southeast side of town near MILK Boulevard, which I would eventually be able to purchase for my mother. Initially Sophia made the down payment on the lease agreement. About one year later I attained employment with a major oil company, and was able to turn our lease into a buy with an additional down payment. Although it was far from perfect, it was better than our previous houses growing up. Helen would cherish the house having birthday dinners for everyone as well as holiday dinners and barbecues. Horace did come by our new place as I continued to keep in contact with him, but we eventually lost contact. I did see him from time to time in passing and learned he eventually married and was divorced. But I remained too busy to keep in contact with anyone.

For a long time I was so busy partying with Becky, whom I met while at the previous office job before acquiring my job at the oil company. We remained club-hopping buddies for the next year. At night Becky worked part time in a liquor store, and was able to get a huge discount, and sometimes she would not even pay. I started to think she had something going with the manager. We would get wasted before we even arrived at the club and whether drunk or sober you better watch your guy around Becky. If she liked him she would go after him, no matter who was dating the guy.

After hanging with Becky I became a party animal. Staying out and always being on the go and meeting different guys just about every few weeks, helped me to forget some of the unhappy and most tragic events of abuse. One night while at the club, Becky introduced me to an acquaintance of one of her friend's. Derrick was very handsome whom I would eventually develop deep feelings. As he treated me with lots of affection along with respect throughout the duration of our relationship, and I fell deeply in love for the first time in my adult life. Derrick and I loved to just sit in the car and kiss. Most of the time we would just end up sitting outside the club kissing. He was a gentleman and never did anything I did not want. After not having a steady boyfriend for a while, I really enjoyed his company although I would eventually find out he was into hard drugs.

One night we decided to meet at Becky's apartment and after we had taken some snapshots in the living room, he started smoking and used her picture frame to cut his white powder. Becky walked in from her bedroom and started yelling. "What the hell do you think your doing on my got damn picture, Derrick, and you know I do not allow any smoking in my house or drug usage. Oh no, you going to have to get the Hell out of here with that, and Nette what is wrong with you. What is he doing to you, you know better than that", she exclaimed as Derrick stormed out of the door. About ten minutes after he left I was lost. I was so out of it, I just stood in her living room very confused. I knew I would never be in that kind of situation again, no mater how much I loved Derrick.

As time passed, I lost contact with Derrick. Then one night I spotted him at a party across the room. To my surprise Becky told me he had gotten married, and I was rather heartbroken to say the least. As I just stood across the room from afar reminiscing of my lost love. I would eventually find out weeks later that he was at a low point in his life, and that's why he married so abruptly. It was partially because his best friend had gotten killed at a nightclub. Becky said it was because Derrick had been trying to talk to some guy's girlfriend. While Derrick only sustained a leg wound, he must have felt horrible as I later found out his best friend was murdered while they were shooting at Derrick. That same night his brother and I started talking, as we dated only a few weeks. I guess I was subconsciously hoping to rekindle the flame with Derrick as I thought it might make him jealous. But it only made things worse. Again my feelings of insecurity and confusion continued to surface as I tried to hide my feelings by overindulging in liquor and dating. Becky advised I should not be dating Derrick's brother, as it did not look right, so eventually broke it off but before long I ended up being introduced to yet another guy. One of Becky's boyfriends introduced us. Although Eric seemed to be a cool guy, he just liked to drink a little too much like myself. One night as we all ended unable to drive home, I somehow ended up at Eric's apartment with about three other guys. While Eric was knocked out upstairs snoring, his little brother dragged me into the living room from Eric's bedroom. The same horrible thing had happened once again, I was rapped over and over again by about three guys. Finally Eric woke up and came downstairs from his deep drunken sleep, but it was a little too late. By that time I was completely sober and ended up at the county hospital. They told me they needed names, including the guy I was dating. I was so confused as I started to think it really wasn't Eric's fault because he was in fact sound asleep. I called him from the hospital and said, "I am thinking about filing charges on your brother as well as his friends. But they need your name and address." He merely responded, "Well I wish you wouldn't, but you do whatever you think you need to do Nette. You knew you should not have even been over here." Again I started to feel once again like it was my fault, I mean maybe I had brought this thing on myself once again. It was just like the first time this happened to me, and I got into West's car when I shouldn't have. I always appeared to end up in the wrong place at the wrong time, and as always I just blamed myself. I must have stayed at the hospital for hours before finally leaving just as confused as I had when I came in. I cried and continued to get wasted for the next few years of my life. I had become an alcoholic. Although I did not drink during the day, I made my way to happy hour every night. If I missed happy hour, I caught the clubs at night. I further keep alcohol by the half-gallons to gallons in my apartment in an attempt to drink away my pain and never-ending tears. I knew something had to change after having several different car accidents the day after partying the night before. One accident occurred when my niece was in the car, as her nose went into the windshield and blood was everywhere. I cried for days, as I would sustain a deviated septum and a jaw injury where my jaws sometimes remain stiff as well as the disc pops in and out of place.

⚡ ⚡ ⚡ ⚡ ⚡ ⚡ ⚡ ⚡ ⚡ ⚡

I would continue to go from relationship to relationship looking for someone to make me forget all the pain, but I only made the worst and it would only get worst before it got better. I recall one night after crying my eyes out over all the mistakes I had made, I happen to turn my attention a minister on television. As he spoke on the pains of life I felt touched as he asked the audience to accept Jesus Christ in their heart and repeat after him. "Jesus I need you to take control over my life, I can't handle it by myself, please come into my life, and I accept you Jesus as my Lord and Savior. Forgive me of my sins and come into my heart, soul, body, and mind. Please change me and make me a new person in the name of Jesus I pray, amen." As I would repeat the prayer I felt liberated having given my life over to Jesus, but I would no doubt have to make a few more mistakes before I would truly grasp the concept of salvation. I had to come to the realization that God sent his son Jesus as a sacrifice for us. Not because it was a necessity, but because he loved the world so much and to demonstrate that love he sent his son Jesus to empower us and be able to overcome our weaknesses, adversities, and shortcomings as human beings. As Jesus died, it was a manifestation of God the father's power in the flesh to in fact overcome evil with good. As I overcame my drinking and smoking habits and continued to pray that I would not stop fighting for my life back. And for the next few years, it would not be anything short of a miracle considering all the past and as well as the future most unfavorable events.

γγγγγγγγγγγγγγγγγγγγγγγγγγγγγγγγγγγγγ

It would be a few years later before I finally deemed any interest in becoming intimate with someone again. But when I did eventually meet someone, he appeared to be a very different man. He was tall rugged yet tender looking man. Richard had a pronounced look of his Cherokee Indian ancestry. He was six feet tall and kept in shape by jogging daily. I mean he was a rather handsome gentleman, and I was in love from the first time I laid eyes on Richard. He mentioned that he was living with someone but they had broken up, and she and her daughter by a previous marriage were in the process of moving. He further invited me over his place, as he exclaimed he had a Christmas gift for me. I was so excited as I put on my finest dress. When I arrived I was so nervous and he offered me a glass of wine, and we sat and watched the Thriller video. He was so impressed with Michael's moves as we all were. As I recall him raving, "Man, Michael is bad. He actually stands up on toes in this video." As he slowed the tape down several times for me to watch. He further commented on Michael's childish like behavior at the end of the video. Then Richard stated, "Michael never had a chance to actually experience a normal childhood. I mean while other kids his age were outside playing, he was on stage performing." Little did Richard know that I too had some most disruptive incidents in my childhood and well into my adult life.

Finally he handed me the gift he bought and whispered Merry Christmas very softly. Then I slowly opened the gift, as it was beautifully wrapped. It was a large box, and I was so surprised as it was a gift certificate for an upscale clothing store. I was taken away as he softly exclaimed, "I know we just met but you appear to be a very nice young lady and I only hope we can get to know each other better". Then we kissed softly, and I was taken away as I felt a real closeness to Richard. I was so totally nervous I could barely speak whenever we were together, and felt as though I was falling in love all over again. For the first time I thought I had met Mr. Right, he was not only a gentleman but intelligent as well. He continually talked to me about all sorts of things. But as I was still quite young and knew very little about real relationships, so I just tentatively listened. He would eventually break up me, and I ended up most devastated and heartbroken.

A few years later, Richard contacted me again and we started seeing each other once more. First, I tried to find out why the relationship was broken off the first time. Richard said he never knew what or how I felt about him because I never talked very much. But just like the first time we dated, I felt he was my soul mate. And as the person for me, I was determined to make it work this time. This time I would tell him how much I cared about him as well as making myself available whenever he called. I tried so hard to keep our lines of communication open.

One day Richard walked up while I was looking in the mirror, as I noticed his skin tone had a deep reddish hue. As I mentioned that I never noticed his deep tone before and being such an intelligent person, he would formulate one of his detailed explanations. He was always so thorough as he would critique most any situation very intelligently. Richard went on to explain how I had a yellow-orange base from my French ancestry, while he had a reddish-brown base similar to his Cherokee ancestors. I fell in love with his cleverness and gentleness, which gave me enough reason to fall deeply in love with him all over again.  But this time I thought it would be different,  he was not just breaking up from a serious relationship I thought so maybe,  just maybe, this is it.  But after only a few weeks,  he would again advise an ex-girlfriend came back.  He would exclaim with much regret,  "She told me she's pregnant".  I was so hurt and disappointed,  words could not express my anguish over this situation,  and I mean I could not believe this was happening again.  So, I asked him very softly and tearfully, "What are you going to do?  Are going to marry her, or just take care for your child".  "I don't know Nanette, but I don't want to hurt you.  I need to find out if I can make it work and at least be a father to my child".

I was mortified as I would sit in my apartment crying for days. My mother called frequently to give me some bible scriptures, which allowed a bit of relief.

ηηηηηηηηηηηηηηηηη

For weeks immediately following this devastating news I continued to try to see Richard until eventually his next-door neighbor advised he was engaged.  I broke down in tears, crying so hard that his neighbor, Broderick became the strong shoulder to lean on.  We eventually started spending time together, and within a few weeks he asked me to marry him.  Not really realizing I was still vulnerable from the recent relationship with Richard, I just simply responded yes. Broderick knew I was still hurting and very vulnerable because of the breakup with Richard, and took total advantage of this delicate situation. Finally the week of the wedding Broderick told me that maybe he asked me to marry too soon, as I guess his conscious had started to bother him. And possibly Richard advised him of his mostly inappropriate actions. When he advised me we were marrying too soon, I just broke down into an extreme panic attack once again.

We eventually decided to proceed with the wedding, although Broderick knew he was taking advantage of this most volatile situation. We had a very nice wedding, and some ladies at work not only gave me lovely gifts but also helped me plan the wedding. Although the marriage only lasted six months, it seemed like a lifetime of pure hell.

Broderick could not keep a steady job and while he said he was looking for work, he would instead drive around my Audi 5000 all day long drinking and visiting his friends while I was at work. We went to his church on Sunday, and sang at various other churches, as he would play the exact same tune on his electric guitar. We further joined his church and the pastor of this small church had two kids with only about two regular members, a deacon and his wife. I remember one night Broderick asked me to direct a visiting choir who, was singing with us. I felt like a total idiot as I reluctantly motioned my hands as if I knew how to direct a choir. Brod was a big con man that liked to show off. After attending church he would take the car and go out at night, partying and quite possibly taking out other ladies. Finally, I was feed up after an incident occurred in which he picked up one of his ex-girlfriends and her children, while I was in the car. "Babe we just going to give her a ride across town to her mama's. Just be cool she don't have a car, and my baby girl is with her. Just be cool, okay babe". Before I could respond about three small children were running toward my car, with their mother not far behind. Not long after that incident I received an application for life insurance with his name as the beneficiary, as he tried to explain I knew I needed to get out of this most disturbing marriage real fast.

That night an argument pursued after Broderick tried to take my car keys and leave. Then after much of my persistence to go with him, he decided to take me along with him. After arriving at this rather small hole in the wall, I could tell there was probably illegal activity going on such as drug dealings and gambling. As Brod sat me down in the club and proceeded toward the back where a curtain separated the two areas, his sister-in-law walked over. We greeted each other rather cheerfully, but she saw right through me, and saw all the pain I was experiencing all over my face. All she said was what's wrong child, and I broke down into tears. As she continued to talk the tears slowly continued to stream down my face, "Listen, let me tell you a few things. You are a young and beautiful woman without any children. Girl my daughter has a baby, and she'll tell a man where to get off. Life is too short for you to be somewhere with someone you do not want to be with. Ain't nothing holding you back from leaving this relationship. So you know what you need to do, you need to make Nanette happy. Ain't' you tired of trying to make everybody else happy. It's your turn girl, it's time for you to use them and then loose them. Now you be the woman I know you can be girl", as she smiled and walked away. It seemed like she said everything I needed to hear to bring me back into some sense of reality. It seemed as though my mind was temporarily disassociated from my body for the pass several years. Those few words she spoke helped give me regain the fire I needed to fight back, and demand some control over my life. That night I finally started to stand up to Brod, something I had never had the courage or even will to do. As he tried to drive my car, I would not give him the keys, "I'm driving tonight", I said boldly. "What, what did you say girl. I don't know what's your problem, but you'd better give me those damn keys ", as he gave me a horrible look. But that night I had just as much Hell in me as he did and merely responded with the exact same fearlessness, "I said I'm driving, it's my damn car and I'm driving. Now you get out of the way because I'm driving," as I looked him straight back in the eye. Brod slowly got out and I crossed over to the driver's seat. I guess I shocked him, I know I did because I shocked myself. The quiet, timid, and frightened little girl finally started to grow up a little bit.

The separation seemed to last as long as the marriage. I would move out and then return, as he and his friends tried to talk me out of leaving. A final deciding factor came when we received a visit from my mother, Helen. One morning she just showed up most unexpectedly. We were both shocked at her visit, she had never really just came over unannounced anywhere, so needless to say I would be listening very assiduously. Helen spoke very firmly saying, "I didn't come to stay long, and I just need to talk to you all about this situation. This going back and forth is no good. Now listen, either you all are going to be together or separate. And Nanette you have put all the furniture in storage saying you have left Brod, but you are still here and sleeping on the floor. What are you doing? Now you need to pray and ask God for guidance because he is not pleased with this situation", and as she left I left with her. It was as though my thinking was clouded as if I was spellbound, but Helen's words along with her prayers somehow broke through it. Within days, I packed up the last of my things and advised the apartment manager I had vacated the premises.

φφφφφφφφφφφφφφφφφφφφφφφφφφφφφφφ

I moved back with Helen, as I wanted to continue to help her as best I could, and wanted to finish paying off the house we purchased. So within a few weeks, I would try to trade in my car for a less expensive model. I needed extra money, so I felt maybe I could get a more reasonable deal. Little did I know the dealership would want me to pay for my car plus the cost of the cheaper car. I soon found out that most cars retain very limited or rather no equitable value.

As I was leaving the car lot in discuss, a tall huge man approached me. He was about six foot three and two hundred pounds, I thought he was kinda handsome. Now I am five feet and no inches, but somehow he felt I might be a match. Joe introduced himself and as we talked, he advised me to just keep my car. Then after some small talk, he asked for my phone number as I advised I was in the middle of a divorce. Needless to say he walked away from my car with my phone number as he stated he was currently going through a divorce as well.

After we talked for a few weeks, he advised me how much trouble his soon to be ex-wife was giving him. Joe said as they were dating she just moved in, and they were married within a few weeks. He further advised how she loved to fight with him, and had slashed his tires and seats of his Mercedes. He advised he would be so glad when this was over, as he visited me often and told me his sad stories. But one night not long after my divorce was final, he came by and we ended up in a heated passion. Within the next few weeks, I was expecting. I was literally in shock as I was twenty-six years old and after six months of marriage had never gotten pregnant, but now I am with child after one night. I guess I had been complacent and rather ill informed in terms of dating and relationships.

But as I thought back over my life and recalled only a few months after breaking up with Richard how I had contemplated suicide as well as experiencing a horrid marriage, I felt this pregnancy was definitely a God sent. This great miracle literally saved my life, and I knew he would be a beautiful baby boy. This strange turn of events gave me a whole new meaning of life and made it worth living again.

As we discussed the situation and he informed me, "I do not believe in abortion. It's killing babies, and I will not be a part of that. I mean I am going to be there for you, because I love you and want to do the right thing." Then he gave me a soft tender kiss on the cheek, which was the last time I saw him during my entire pregnancy. Subconsciously I thought his actions did not bother me, because I knew I would have enough love and everything else our son might need. But deep within my very soul was a hurt that only could be repaired by nothing short of a mere miracle from God.

During the entire pregnancy when I would lye down I exhibited extreme difficulty breathing due to my small frame, as I would feel the baby literally pushing in my chest or lung area. My pregnancy was rather intense when I had to sleep in an upright position on the sofa, with my feet stretched out. I further developed fibroid tumors but through all the difficulties, I was just about the happiest pregnant lady there was considering my condition. I continually took pictures before and after Joseph's birth, he was in fact a beautiful baby. As most of my picture taking was after his birth, and I would write a corky caption underneath each one of his pictures which included his age for the first few months. I further ordered cake decorating books and supplies, as I desired to do beautiful homemade cakes and candies for his birthdays as well as holidays. I was so entrepreneurial I even did a few for family and friends, which soon became overwhelming. But I continued to enjoy taking care of my bundle of joy, as I steamed and pureed fresh vegetables daily. Joseph loved the steamed broccoli with cheese sauce, as well as carrots, cauliflower, and other vegetables. Also, I made sure he had his daily dose of polyvisol liquid vitamins. I tried to keep myself occupied from remodeling the floors to reading during my pregnancy, and in the meantime I found out how important proper nutrition was to the development of the fetus and newborn. Even today I still try to make sure my son takes a good multiple vitamin and eats right, while trying to exclude lots junk food such as soda, gum, certain candies, chips, and foods with preservatives and artificial flavors and coloring.

☺ er er er er er er er er er er er

Joe finally called the night of my delivery date, as I believe the stress finally got to me. That night my water broke as soon as I hung up the phone. The doctor decided to give me a caesarian after about twelve hours of labor, and Joseph appeared to be incorrectly positioned. I was sick and stayed in the hospital five days, even my jaw was hurting. The doctor said because I had previous TMJ (temporal mandibular joint) jaw problems, air probably seeped into the joint area during the surgery.

✝ ✝ ✝ ✝ ✝ ✝ ✝ ✝ ✝ ✝ ✝ ✝ ✝ ✝ ✝ ✝ ✝ ✝

Joe showed up at the hospital the next day. Just in time to see his son, his cousin came with him and exclaimed, "Man that baby looks just like you Joe." As I later discovered Joe was still married, and his wife was expecting as we conceived our son. I was devastated as I visited his parents, and his mother was very honest with me and told me everything. He was never going through a divorce like I was, but instead had started what would be years of drug usage. His grandmother further told me he had several other children, and lost his own car dealership business. She further advised Joe turned to drugs after loosing everything.

Joe eventually started to visit his son about every few months, and often times he would try to get money from me. One day he came by, as he said he was divorced from his wife. He stayed a few days and I was tempted once again to believe him, as he was my son's father. I wanted desperately for him to be a father to his son, for I loved my son more than life itself. I wanted my son to have everything all the other children had, and that included a father. But after a few days he left making some ridiculous claim of being angry because I did not name our son, Joseph, after him.

Finally after an empty visit to the his Catholic Church where we discussed marriage once again, he would exclaim he needed some type of form from the priest while still refusing to admit he was married. Finally after stating the priest was not available, he decided to visit his grandmother, and he took my son and I over her house for a few days. I was puzzled as he would normally take us over his mother's, but I later learned his mother had put him out because of his addiction. That night we drove to the corner store where he confronted me about giving him cash again. I refused stating I did not have any money. He went into a rage and started shouting in face, "you got money. You know you got some money and I want it now". I continued to refuse as I was frightened by his rage. He sped off and we went back to his grandmother's house. Then after a few moments he walked back over toward my purse and before I knew it, he grabbed my keys and sped off in my car again. I did not here from Joe until that next afternoon, he said he was bringing me the car. The next time I saw my car was in the wrecking yard totally stripped. The seats, locks, tires, and even the clothes I had in the trunk that I was taking to the cleaners were all gone. All was left was a pair of my dress shoes, and they were mashed and dirty. As I looked on the situation heartbroken and filled with despair I could not believe my eyes. I later found out why his mother put him out, because he stole and stripped her car as well. I guess it slipped her mind, because she failed to mention that to me. Afterwards I tried to file charges, but the district attorney refused. He then just continued to be incarcerated in attempt to support his habit. As I pray one day he would be saved.

As my son became school age, he would often ask why he did not have a father like other children. I recall one day while driving him home from school he announced, "I want a Daddy. Look there's a guy

walking right over there. He can be my Daddy." I eventually learned his
teacher was asking the students about their father's. I immediately went
to the principal as I thought it was most inappropriate behavior. I was
heartbroken over my son's desire to have a family, as I knew I wanted
and needed it for him as well. Eventually I started to date again hoping
to build the family my son wanted, but after a series of more bad
relationships I was more messed up than ever before. Finally after not
hearing from Joe for over ten years, one day I received a call, "Well
Hello Ms. Bruneaux". I was stunned as I asked, "Who is this"? "This is
Joe".

"Joe, How did you get this number", I exclaimed.

"I just called the company's main switchboard and asked for your
number."

"How's Joseph".

As I replied slowly, "He's okay. I can't believe how you can just leave
your son without even one call Joe."

Joe continued to respond, "I know and all I can do is say I'm sorry. I
just want to talk to him. Can I call him if you don't mind".

"I don't know Joe. It's been ten years. Joseph does not even remember
you."

"I mean I know I haven't been there, but I just want to talk to him."

As he continued to call me, I eventually gave him the home phone
number. I had spoken with Joseph on several occasions about his father's
phone calls and how he wanted to talk, as I received virtually no
response from Joseph. When his father would call and ask to speak to
him, Joseph would just refuse to come to the phone. One time he pulled
the phone back from my ear to listen to his voice, but continued his
refusal to talk with his father. As I was right in the middle of the
controversy, Joe began to accuse me of not letting him talk to his son. I
continued to encourage Joseph to express his feelings whether positive or
negative. But as I encouraged him to voice his feelings, he finally wrote
his father a letter asking his father why he left. Joseph was merely
looking for some answers. As Joseph never received a response, I
became enraged, "Why haven't you replied to Joseph's letter." Joe

responded, "I call almost everyday and he doesn't want to talk and besides I think you wrote that letter not Joseph. You know you could make that boy come to the phone if you wanted too."

I exclaimed, "I cannot believe you Joe. If you were serious about building a relationship with your son, you would do whatever you had to do and that is responding to his letter. Furthermore, Joseph is almost twelve years old and he has feelings. What do you think? Just because he is young he doesn't know anything. He has feelings. I have barely talked about you to Joseph, but he knows you have not been there for him. He knows I love him because I am here taking care of him, he does not know if you even care. You need to give this child more credit and stop blaming me for your mistakes. Joe, you never even once visited or even taken care of your son.

Joseph wrote yet one more letter as he asked his father why didn't he respond to the first letter. As I had once again asked him to make some attempt to respond to his son's letter, within a few days after I talked to his mother, Joe was back out on the street. I don't know if he ever saw the second letter from Joseph. Within a manner of weeks he was back in jail for theft, and about a couple of years later he was still in jail. At that time I laid in hospital having fibroid tumors removed, I later learned Joe's grandmother passed the same day I had surgery. I recall the last time Joseph and I went to see his great grandmother just a few weeks before she would pass, she had a real bad cough and spoke of how her brother had just passed. As her house was filled with second hand smoke, I would just advise her to try to eat right and she agreed while handing Joseph five dollars. She was always trying to give Joseph something, and further trying to get her family together to see her great-grandson, Joseph. She would ask me to come over and have a party for Joseph as his grandfather had a horse ranch, but I never did and I sometimes regret it. I was also afraid of what Joe might do as he was still fighting his addiction, and I still had ill feeling for his actions, which included neglecting his son.

I guess deep down inside I never got over Joe's actions. Still inwardly grieving about Joseph's father as my life began to continue take a bad turn. Yet still quite trusting and fooling myself into thinking I would never be vulnerable again. But it happened yet again not long after Joe had decided to steal my car. It seemed like I could never give myself time to heal from life's travesties.

✿✿✿✿✿✿✿✿✿✿✿✿✿✿✿✿✿✿✿

I recall when my son, Joseph, was still rather small just a few days after Joe had taken my car, I met a guy that I thought could help make the family Joseph and I longed for. After dating him for a while, I finally realized how I was really over my son's father, Joe. It took me a long time to realize his true intentions were very different than mine, as I further recall being on muscle relaxants for months due to the jaw pain from my first auto accident. I started to overuse these prescription drugs, as I took twice the prescribed dosage. I guess that was why I could not regain my composure, and it took me over two years to realize this was not the guy for me. This older more experienced man met me at a low point in my life, and he was neither the role model nor the husband I needed. He once even told me I should give my son away to my sister. He further told me he could not have children, and not long after I found myself pregnant. He said, "You must have been pregnant from Joe your previous boyfriend." The next time he claimed, "Something must have changed because my doctor told me I could not have kids." He advised it couldn't happen again. The next time I got pregnant I begged him not to abort our baby but he responded, "What do you want with a crumb snatcher?" I knew this was not meant to be as the doctor further stated once again that the baby was almost gone anyway, which was not surprising considering his sometimes unduly and sometimes rough behavior at times. I knew my search for a husband and father for my son was not going anywhere, and none of this was meant to be. I then tried to forget all the painful relationship mistakes, and returned to my first and most important dream of achieving a college education.

I had previously attended Texas Southern University right after high school and majored in Journalism part-time, and only needed thirty college hours for the degree.  At the time I was a most undecided freshman as I changed my mind on my major a few times.  While growing up I wanted to be a medical doctor after my Dad died of a fatal heart attack.  By high school it was a psychology,  but I eventually choose my first love, writing. TSU did not have offer creative writing classes at the time and I ended up majoring in Journalism. I recall getting bored in one of my communications courses and I just left the class.  As I sat outside I just started to write, as I desperately needed to be in a creative writing course.

〰〰〰〰〰〰〰〰〰〰

As I finally returned after my son was born majoring in Journalism was no longer an option, I had wasted too much time.  This last relationship kept me out once again totaling about four years that I did attend college.

As I returned to school once again after Joseph was born, but this time was different.  Joseph was my inspiration, and main reason for continuing my dreams.  So this time I decided not to waste time dating, and I would discontinue the medication and try to heal my body naturally.  After a couple of years I was able to graduate from University of Houston with a Bachelors in Business, and a concentration in Computer Information Systems.  This was no doubt a far cry from my original degree plans, but I would finally achieve my childhood dream of being a college graduate, which was nothing short of a miracle.  It was a bittersweet reality as Helen's health started to deteriorate the same summer I received the long awaited honor of receiving a college degree. It was the summer of 1994, the summer my dear mother, Helen would stop walking.

Chapter 6: 'Helen's Fall'

Helen loved attending church and strongly believed in God, and she loved her family just as much. Helen put her own interest and health on the back burner to care for others. I remember how she and Daddy would care for my niece as a baby, and once Daddy passed she was left to carry the load. But Helen loved to baby-sit the grandchildren, while she would unknowingly neglect her health.

She eventually developed severe rheumatoid arthritis basically due to a fall she suffered while mopping one of the many rooms at work. After going to their doctor, it was determined she was not injured even though several of her fingers appeared badly bent and remained crooked or rather dislocated. Also, her left knee was badly swollen, as all injuries remained noticeable and would only worsen as the years passed. This fall occurred not long before my father passed away, and my father would often say we would do a lot better if he were dead as he looked at his VA disability pension. But that became an unreasonable untruth, as Helen would eventually have to quit working at the YMCA as she became unable to stand for long periods of time. She suffered stomach problems from the taking arthritis medications. Finally one of her doctor's suggested replacing her kneecap, but Helen was adamantly against removing or replacing any of her body parts. She almost appeared to be fearful with the thought of any type of medical procedure or surgery. I felt this stemmed from her childhood experiences with physicians as well as some of her siblings early deaths.

Helen spoke of when she was younger how the doctors would be out after nightfall looking for people to experiment on. She talked of how the people in white jackets roamed around at night looking for unsuspecting people to capture by hitting them over the head. Once captured the person would eventually end up in the morgue, as you would never hear from them again. She would also often talk about Junior, the nephew she raised, and how she saw the doctors cut open his head for experimentation purposes. From hearing stories as a child to living in an unpredictable world as an adult, Helen developed a real and unending fear of doctors. And I suppose it was rightfully considering all the tragedy, and most untimely deaths she experienced with her relatives.

Now this unending fear was unfolding in her life, after her last hospital visit when she had become a near paraplegic. Although she could still move her hands and arms, her arthritic knee would not allow her to walk very well, as she would fall numerous times. The doctors said all the cartilage in the knee had deteriorated, and it was bone rubbing against bone. I could only imagine what excruciating pain my mother was experiencing. One day while walking she fell and slammed her head into the wall loosing consciousness. Her condition was really bad as she was also diagnosed with congestive heart failure, high blood pressure, and diverticulitis to name a few. She could not eat any corn, seeds, nuts, or and any roughage as they would puncture the polyps from the diverticulitis cause profuse bleeding. Between her bad knee and diverticulitis she would faint while walking, as she would bleed from her rectum and mouth simultaneously.

As Helen's condition worsened, I knew poor previous and current diet was not helping this situation either. As I was aware of some nutrition and disease correlation, but there had to be something more as I tried dig deeper to further understand her situation. Still unable to fully grasp the concept, I needed more information on this matter. In an effort to further my understanding, I ordered a book on Arthritis and per this reading I gave Helen high doses of vitamin C and E along with a multivitamin I purchased from a local store. The high dosage of vitamin C was too acidic and Helen's lips would swell from all the acid. Fearing the effect of this high dosage I discontinued giving it to her. At this time I did not have very much information about vitamins, aging, arthritis, or general health for that matter.

Then one day while my mother babysat my sister's daughter, she fell once again. This fall would be devastating as it rendered her unable to walk, and literally dependent on others for all her personal needs. My mother now required twenty-four hour care. As I would always move back and forth to the house I purchased for Helen as all her children, but this time I thought maybe the rest of my family would probably feel the need to help out more.  My sisters advised they would take care of Helen, but after a couple of weeks they decided to put her into a private home for the elderly.

After watching her suffer for about a week in this private home, I decided to take her back to her house.  I could not bear seeing her not eating as she had become depressed, and very frail from this move.  I felt if she stayed in that place one more day, she would probably die soon. So I hired a nurse aid and we picked her up, and took Helen back home.

I paid nurses to care for my mother almost twenty-fours hours a day. Then as I went bankrupt, I called my eldest brother, Fred.  He agreed to move in with Helen and care for her.  I thought everything was working well until one Sunday afternoon, our family ties started to wreak havoc.

Fred had asked my sister, Velma, to come over and stay with Helen as he was going to be gone for most of the day.  As Velma was caring for Helen, she received a phone call that Hortense, her birth mother and Helen's niece, had passed away in Dallas.  Velma continued to care for Helen that day along with that sad news, as well as dealing with her marital and family problems of her own.

When I arrived I was shocked to find Fred and Velma arguing profusely, as the pressure of our failing mother's health started to take its toll on this very close nit family bond.  As I tried to settle the situation down to no avail, and was in total disbelieve as I watched my family who I saw withstand the most difficult of difficult times fall apart.  Finally, I walked outside for moment and when I returned Fred and Velma were in a scuffle.  Fred had his arm wrapped around Velma, as it appeared she was biting his arm.  It was most disturbing situation and rather heart wrenching as two most loving siblings were now embarked in physical a brawl.  Fred left the house that day and only returned to pick up his belongings.  But now as I look back and think about the situation, it looked pretty comical, because neither one of them wished to hurt each other.  They were just venting their frustration, although it was most unfortunate.

Not long afterwards, Helen legs started to swell profusely as pockets of pus developed.  I called for the ambulance and they diagnosed her situation, and just as they were going to release her I advised the hospital there was no one at the house to care for her as work during the day. They agreed to keep her in a special transitional unit, and tried to council with the family as no one ever showed up for the meetings. Finally, as they were about to discharge her Velma advised she would be moving in with Helen. Velma further found a live-in sitter Monday through Friday for Helen.

Then after a few weeks passed, Velma settled her marital problems and went back to her home. As her daughter needed a place to stay, she moved in with Helen. She took pretty good care of Helen for a while, but as she let some of her friends move in and after Helen's second hospital visit, I decided to move Helen out the house. I put her into a facility recommended by her doctor. He advised that although it was a long-term care facility, they would be able to provide physical therapy and possibly regain her mobility. This sounded like the best option as I thought they could help Helen walk again, but as time passed things took a turn for the worst.

Helen was so unhappy there, as I had to visit her daily to make her eat. As I visited I became accustom to a strong scent, which was similar to a baby' soiled diaper. I further noticed small holes in the floor where ants were coming into the room. I was so worried I visited Helen sometimes twice a day stressing to the facility how they needed to close the holes. I even tried to cover the holes, as I would take masking tape with me while visiting my mother. I later learned an elderly person did die from ant bites, I could only imagine it was in the same room my mother was in. I would stop at the drug store and pick up her nutritional drinks and take it to her on my lunch breaks. I even moved in a house not far from the facility in order to cut my driving time. There were times when I felt overwhelmed and as I would try to pray, all I could say was Jesus. Sometimes just repeating the name of Jesus over and over again while driving over twenty miles to and from my job to visit and care for my mother.

As I pressured the facility increase her physical therapy and move her to another room, they advised she had reached her maximum level of recovery. And as they resisted my request to move her, I continued to exclaim she could not walk and they were running the risk of her dying if left in a room with ants. Finally after a few weeks, they moved Helen to another room. Not long after her move, I started planning on taking Helen back home. But before I reached that point I received a call about three o'clock in the morning, apparently Helen had fallen from the bed. I rushed over to the emergency room and all I could do was pray that Helen would be okay. I sat just and waiting for all her tests to return, as they stitched up her head injury. After a few hours the hospital said nothing was broken or damaged, but over the next few weeks I watched her leg slowly start to draw up. As I read the report from the facility, I became more and more suspicious. As the facility insisted Helen climbed over the rail and fell to the floor, I knew the story was not a wash. My mother was not able to move herself, nor was she capable of lifting her body over a bed rail. Helen could barely move on her own ability. After talking with a couple of the workers, they admitted a partially paraplegic aide had dropped her while putting her in bed.

Immediately following this fall, Helen told me about another incident that happened in the home. She spoke of being tied up and was still sore as they pulled the string between her private areas. I was devastated and knew I had to get her out of there and fast.

While in the facility Helen's previous roommate's daughter followed her stay, as she took a special interest in my mother's situation. She would always visit with Helen whenever she came, and even gave Helen some pictures of her family. She further knew my dilemma and that Helen did not want to be there, as well as how I did not want her there any longer. She finally told me about a new program that the states human resources department had recently approved. The program provided a few more hours than the other state programs. This would allow me to provide care for Helen while at work.

Although they accepted Helen into the program, there was a waiting list. I advised the social worker of Helen's bad experiences in the home and as she was most sympathetic to our delicate situation. Immediately after the fall I called the social worker again in order to speed up the process for Helen's return home. The social worker was very understanding and advised, "under the circumstances, I will see what I can do to expedite the process", within a few weeks she agreed to hire a caregiver the same day I would bring Helen home. Finally, all I needed to get my mother out of this home was to locate a state certified agency to admit her into their company with a caregiver. I immediately started to search for a caregiver calling all the local employment agencies, churches, or anybody that I felt could help. They were very understanding and within a short period of time I had packed up Helen things and we were on our way back home.

That day when I returned home with Helen, Velma's daughter was still living in the house, but moved out a few days later. My nephew stayed there with my mother a few weeks, until I moved in while waiting for our new house to be finished. I had previously invested in some country property, as I originally wanted to build a country home after my son was born. I was tired of apartments and now my agenda had to be changed as I felt I needed a place not only for my son, and myself but for my mother as well. Helen needed twenty four-hour assistance, and I now knew I had to be the person to take over that responsibility. It was certain I did not want to live in the same house where all the tragedy occurred, so I decided to sell my country property, opting to build instead, in an existing subdivision since it would be ready fairly quickly.

Another deciding factor for me to takeover the care for Helen, besides the unsafe environment of that nursing home was it was just a natural that I continue to look after her. Not to mention the mess I continued to make in my life. While I decided to bring Helen home I was dating a man who was an Educator. He seemed to be descent man with two adult daughters and a grandson, and appeared to be the perfect father figure for Joseph. As our relationship progressed and I continued to worry about Helen, I negligently ended up pregnant once again. He demanded I have an abortion, as he finally would admit to me he had another ten-year-old daughter. I debated his demands for weeks contemplating how I would take care of a child that the father did not want, because I knew this should not be happening now. After long and tiring conversation with a most unyielding man, I regretfully agreed since I would never trap a person into a relationship. Immediately following the horrible experience I was sick and depressed, and that same night I began to write the introduction to this book, Choices for the Choiceless, as I sat writing trying to feel comfort, but to no avail. Once again crying so long and hurting so deeply from another ridiculous mistake in my confused life. It seemed like not only did I have bad judge of character, but also I always ended up in unwarranted situations. As I had been consumed with making sure Helen was cared for, I would somehow loose control of my biological clock. And although my mother did not encourage premarital bliss, she did reiterate if one us did find ourselves in an intimate situation to always get up immediately afterwards. I felt there could probably be some validity this statement since all of my siblings were a few years apart, and the last three of us all almost exactly two years apart. What was wrong with me? As I knew I needed to start leading a more fulfilling life. I was raised not to embrace premarital bliss, as it was not only a sin against God but also not his will in my life. Therefore, I finally decided to abstain over the few years. I had been celibate before, and intimacy was not a driving force for my existence. I had made far too many mistakes and just maybe living my life alone, which excluded premarital bliss, would prove to be a wise decision. I felt God was trying to tell me this was not his will, and one would think by now I would know better. But it was not a matter of logic, but in fact deep routed psychological events in my life just like the tragic molestation as a child and events of the rape almost twenty years ago. While I always thought I wanted to be married, I was so insecure. I actually subconsciously felt that I did not deserve to be married in the mist of making poor judgment calls, and possibly dating the wrong guys. I could not think reasonably when it came to love, intimacy, and how it all fits together with relationships and in fact I went into the relationships foreseeing it would fall apart.

Not long after this catastrophe, I met a minister who became a good friend. He was a man of God and tried to assist me in looking for houses before I decided to finally build. As I wanted Joseph to stay in his current school district, but I wanted to move from my current apartment into a house a house with a yard. After searching for this new house almost every weekend, I finally decided to build, but in time this house would soon prove an unwise choice as well.

We moved into the house with from my brother, and my newly found friend who desired to marry immediately. But I was too overwhelmed by my past, so he moved on with his quest for his wife and children. It appeared as though God had finally put what I wanted in my lap, but I needed time to try and get over all my pain, and become a woman who could honestly love herself, as I did not like me very much. Hence, I decided to move forward with contentment as I needed to do a different and hopefully right thing, and that was providing care for my aging mother and raise my son with God's help.

Buying a house would be conducive to Joseph needs, as well as Helen's most delicate condition was also my main objective. Joseph would get the stairs he always wanted as well as be able to attend a good school. Helen needed a larger bedroom as well as a bathroom that would be wheelchair assessable. This house proved to be an ill-informed decision as I ended up without a bedroom and full bath downstairs, we had so needed. The sales person talked me into an existing floor plan, in which I could turn the downstairs study into my mother's bedroom. Furthermore although Joseph acquired the stairs he requested, and I had the bedroom downstairs for Helen we still had continuing problems with the workmanship. I eventually decided to try and sue the builder as he consistently refused to repair the problems correctly, but my lawyer would receive most of the compensation. But I decided not to dwell on the negative and just deal with the situation as best I could, and concentrate on the positive aspects while counting my blessings.

As Joseph loved his new school and did well in his core classes, I further encouraged him to move toward sports or music as for his extracurricular activities to help occupy his mind. But he vowed to take French every year as his extracurricular activity. As I supported and encouraged his actions, I too loved French as I had taken it my first year in high school. No doubt I am proud of Joseph and of his zest for life and learning. I guess although we did not know any of our ancestors, there was a part of our souls that profoundly overwhelmed all the negatives, as he desired to learn everything about them. His attitude is positive and he exhibits love for all people, and he attempts to correct me if I make reference to a Black person as sister or if reference anyone's race he responds, "Why are you talking about someone's race. Mom, it doesn't matter, people are people." Of course I have taught him to love everyone and now he is only following my lead very well, as he has learned to pick apart my every word. The bad thing about his nagging was I really did not mean any harm as I sometimes may describe an individual by their color, but I am glad he keeps me from sounding like I might. My son is the new generation and can only hope they have profoundly missed the curse of racism, as he loves everyone so freely honestly. He reminds me of myself, as I appeared to be the only one to denounce race in my newly desecrated school, as I made friends with all races of people. He further revealed to me his desire to remove racial profiling questionnaires from every phase of our society, as he feels we are all one human race. He feels there is not a justification for a race based our society, but rather it should be strictly based on merit. Although I agree with his ideas, I further had to advise him he must devise ways to eliminate the face-to-face practices before final decisions are made, as our eyes sometimes subconsciously may make these decisions. But his ideas are most compelling and brilliant.

Having my son Joseph as well as caring for my mother was no doubt my chance to do something right, I had made so many mistakes and sometimes continued to make them daily. But now I am raising a loving son and caring for a person who would otherwise might not even be alive. But maybe just maybe in the mist of my totally confused life I could do something good for someone else. It was no longer about my warped self-absorbed decisions, but it was about helping another, who happened to be my mother and my son. I could only pray that within the process I might find a healing for myself from the past abuse, and that this would be a start a new wiser me in life.

As we made the transition to the new house, my oldest brother Fred moved most of the furniture from the old house.  When we first moved into the new house, Fred and his wife continued to provide some daily care for my mother's as Fred had previously helped out.  In the following weeks I would have to find a new caregiver within this new part of town, as my brother had other obligations.  I recall mentioning to some coworkers about how I was having problems finding a caregiver for my mother, then after much prayer from everyone we found a wonderful Christian lady.  Rachel was God sent as she cared for my mother everyday.  Rachel even came in to care for Helen when she was sick, just out the goodness of her heart and love for my mother.

*"Be not overcome of evil.... but overcome evil with good"*
                                                          *Romans*

Chapter 7:  The Healing Quest Begins:
    *'As Knowledge Revels from Lessons Learned Almost*
        *But Not Too Late'*

        After not walking for almost a year, Helen's muscles began to stiffen and become contracted, and if you moved her in the wrong way she would screech in pain.  For a long time I harbored lots of guilty feelings.  If I had only known or had paid closer attention to this most delicate situation, maybe she would not have been so bad off.  I feel partially responsible and desired to do something, just anything to make this most gloomy situation better.
Consequently an extraordinary thing happened one day while at work in the mid-*1996*:  One of my coworkers shared a book with me about herbs. Within a manner of moments the healing quest began.  I had been frequently talking about my mother 's illness and as this lady brought her book on herbs, sometimes I often wonder if she actually knew the how much she helped.  Not only did this book contain a wealth of information, but also it empowered me as I started feeling more in control of this most new and difficult situation.  After absorbing as much information as possible from the book and other mustered information, I made my way to the health food store where I would eventually purchase a couple of books.  This was my answer once again from God as I began to feel more in control.
        I could not stop myself as I had previously read a few books on arthritis and home remedies, but this new information was very different. Eventually we started to visit the health food stores on our lunch break. At first I bought a couple of books and referenced the copies we had made and started Helen on an herbal treatment program, but eventually acquired a lot more books, magazines, and other information from various sources.  This new knowledge gave me a deeper understanding of the human body as I even learned history of some plants including herbs in their entirety.  It further taught me how chemically treated or partially modified foods are not as nutritionally sound as the complete or rather whole food.

At the time I started this quest Helen was taking all sorts of medications. Medications such as antidepressants, arthritis painkillers, and pills increase her appetite, and pills to help her sleep at night. I watched as my mother sometimes hallucinated and other times seemed lethargic, while the muscles as well as tissues in her whole body continued to deteriorate.

As she would often times stay awake all night long hallucinating from the antidepressants along with all the other medications. Helen's system was so toxic and out of balance she could have departed a long time ago. After taking various medications, not eating properly, and partially incapacitated, Helen stayed impacted along with continuous bedsores.

Finally, after watching her continue to suffer I decided to take her off all the arthritis medications that caused the stomach problems. Also, I took her off the sleeping pills, the antidepressants, and the appetite pills. At the time I took her off these medications, as she was not taking anything vital to her well being such as a heart medication or any other health threatening disease. For her arthritis, corticosteroid medications were prescribed such as injections or oral forms, which was short term relieve for the pain. She took these medications and overtime the long-term use of these medications called non-steroidal anti-inflammatory (NSAID's) drugs, which would temporarily relieve her arthritic pain, can result in other problems including adrenal cortex disorders such as Cushing's Syndrome. Adrenal glands are a part of the endocrine system that produces hormones, which includes the pituitary glands, thyroid and parathyroid, the pancreas as well as the reproductive organs. The adrenal gland produces the hormones for proper body functions from regulating blood pressure and metabolizing, to regulating stress. Your own bodies over production of cortisol hormone due to disease, poor nutrition, smoking, drug abuse and too much stress, or the cortisone drugs can lead to the characterization of Cushing's Syndrome. This disease can be treated to help normalize cortisol production by prescribing non-corticosteroid drugs for pain, and other prescription drugs can be prescribed to reduce cortisol. In some cases if the

Cushing's relates to a tumor on the pituitary gland it can be treated with radiation and these treatments can cause other hormone deficits and can be treated by hormone replacement, but leaving Cushing's syndrome untreated can lead to other illness and eventual death. Symptoms of overproduction of cortisol can include eye problems such as cataracts, weight gain, rounding of the face, diabetes, and high blood pressure. Further resulting in thinning bones, muscles, and some skin brusing. Although my mother was never tested for Cushing's, she did exhibit most if not all of the symptoms. Her muscles and bones started wasting away as well as her thin skin resulted in bruising. She further exhibited the enlarged hump at the back of her neck at the beginning of the spin area, along with problems healing.

But unquestionably the long-term usage of these arthritic medications started to erode her stomach lining causing ulcers, and other associated digestive problems. She eventually acquired a gastrologist as her primary care physician, as Helen started to literally just chew up her food and spit the fiber substance back out. Finally her throat was literally closing up from all the NSAID's arthritic medications, her doctor had to periodically perform a dilation procedure enabling her to swallow the fiber portion of the food again.

I further learned that some arthritis or inflammatory symptoms could be associated with a tick bite, which develops into Lyme disease. Also arthritic symptoms can develop from an untreated bacterial infection such as gonococcus or staph. All these conditions can lead to joint swelling and destruction, which we now call arthritis. Some of the treatments I found for rheumatoid arthritis included antibiotic treatment, as some believe this in a mycoplasma infection. Diseases modifying anti-rheumatic drugs (DMARDs) are affiliated with the antibiotic family of drugs. An example of DMARDs is Minocycline (Minocin) which is in the family of tetracycline's have been prescribed with pain relievers. As these drugs are slow acting and take a few months to show benefits, some believe early detection and treatment with prescribing tetracycline antibiotics can thereby prevent the progression the disease. While others believe progression of this disease, that results in destruction to the joints is no doubt inevitable.  But no matter the treatment, it was certain that my mother at the age of seventy-eight was well into the degenerative phase of this disease.

    After realizing these facts surrounding rheumatoid arthritis as an autoimmune disease I started to treat it with a multiple vitamins, minerals, and herbs, which naturally boost the immune system.  The 'immune system' help fight off toxins, which may invade our body through bad food, bad water, and pollution.  But an autoimmune disease is where the body actually destroys itself as it no longer recognizes or differentiates between toxins and good tissues and quite simply destroys good cells.

Nutritional Notes:

    The first herbs I used for her digestive problems consisted of *acidophilus*, which builds and replaces the bad intestinal bacteria with good intestinal flora.  I further mixed one part *aloe vera* juice with one part *apple juice* that removes heavy metal toxins, and included dandelion for a needed cleansing program. Aloe vera juice which helps cell regeneration, heals skin disorders, stomach and digestive disorders, and *dandelion* cleanses the blood, liver, reduces cholesterol, uric acid, improves kidney functions, pancreas, spleen, stomach, anemia, boils, abscesses, tumors, cirrhosis of the liver, hepatitis, jaundice, rheumatism, fluid retention, age spots, and breast cancer. Dandelion as well as *milk thistle* or wild artichoke helps autoimmune diseases. Milk thistle also helps protect and rebuild the liver from further damage and beneficial for adrenal gland disorders. **Wheat germ** derived from wheat berry lowers cholesterol and is a good source of fiber and vitamin E.

    Also made her a wonderful cleansing soup, in which Helen stated it was similar to the soups her mother would make when she was a child. The soup included lots of *parsley* which helps the liver, bladder, lung, stomach, thyroid functions, digestive system, relieves gas and indigestion, expels worms, fluid retention, halitosis, high blood pressure, kidney disease and functions, prostate disorders, contains substances that inhibit tumor growth, and high in vitamin C.

    Other soup ingredients included celery, *onion* (fight tumor growth), *garlic* (antibiotic properties), beets, kale (cruciferous vegetable good for the colon and fight colon cancer), greens, and a small turnip which I found sometimes gave the soup a slightly bitter taste hence I always added half distilled water and half organic apple juice. Organic fruits and vegetables are grown with stricter guidelines, hence I started to buy organic as often as possible. The apple juice tended to give the soup a slighter smoother taste in which Helen was accustom too, since my mother would normally add sugar to every dish she cooked. Sometimes I included all natural meat or soup bones, and further attempted to completely eliminate all preservatives from our diet. I had read and became familiar with the toxic affects of these harmful substances such as preservatives on the fetus during my pregnancy. Preservatives such as monosodium glutamate or nitrates, which may be included some meats and various foods. I further always read the label and shopped only for natural products and natural food stores. Also eliminating colors and dyes from our foods as well. I added plenty of garlic, which has been known to have natural antibiotic properties, as well as a heart formulated garlic capsule with cayenne pepper, vitamin E, and hawthorn berries. Believe it or not cayenne pepper is good for stomach problems such as ulcers.

*Late 1997-1998*

I made sure I kept fresh fruit and vegetable juice, and although it was rather time consuming sometimes, I utilized my lunch breaks to stop by the health food store. And Rachel or I would take her outside to attain some needed sunlight for her healing. Sunlight provides vitamins for healing the inner body. While Helen had minor bedsores quite often, I had acquired a lot of help the first couple of years. The nursing agencies would come out and sometimes help me feed her dinner and ready for bed. As they tried to put her to bed she would sometimes end up right back in her recliner. Helen hated lying straight as she said it made her arthritic knee hurt worst. Initially she started sleeping in chairs a few years before my father passed and continued the practice after falling injury at work, which left her virtually unable to lye in bed comfortably. I would purchase her several recliners and the last one I purchased was from the medical supply store. But I continued my efforts to coerce her to lie in bed to no avail, as I would end up having to return her to the recliner sometimes during the middle of the night. Helen could not bear lying down as the pain intensified. As Helen sometimes sat in her chair during the day she constantly talked of going places, I am sure deep down inside she wished to be able to go somewhere, but could not. As I watch my mother's anguish surface daily from being unable to walk, I now have even more of a desire to reach every single goal I have set for myself. I can only imagine how depressing it can be to wish to do something and cannot because of a sickness or disease, but I believe my mother's faith is what keep her going through it all. Because deep down inside her soul she knew that Jesus still loved her, as it appeared he provided plenty of care from a lot of loving people around her.

After the visiting skilled nurses and her daytime caregiver, Rachel, had gotten her bedsores under control, the nurse assistants discontinued their visits. Then as the nurses started to discontinue and limit their visits, I asked my siblings to come over and help out on the weekends. As my sisters started coming over on weekends to help with my mother, Sophia asked me to write down what I wanted done for Helen. I felt it might be a good idea to list the information for Helen on a sheet for anyone or in case anyone else besides Rachel had to prepare her vitamin regiment. As I had purchased a vitamin box and started to change and add some combinations, I printed the most current information sheet in the following manner and posted it on the refrigerator:

### Helen's Information/Tasks

*About 8:30AM - First task before cleaning up - 1 or 2 Arthritis capsules with full glass of water. Please note she may only drink a little but try to continue giving her sips of water.*

*Second task - Clean-up/Bathe and put aloe vera lotion on and castor oil on joint and back (helps arthritis stiffness) areas as well as very dry skin areas.*

*9:30 to 10AM - Third - Fix Breakfast - please use egg with soy/rice or almond milk also add all seasonings on stove center. Also note plenty of parsley is good. Toast bread (tapioca or rice bread) put butter mixture in container (parsley, garlic, flax oil, butter or plain yogurt) and jam. If butter mixture not made, use olive oil as well as apple butter. One-cup herbal antioxidant tea combination.*

*Fourth - Give vitamin juice labeled 'All One' or if not made please make juice while eating. Mix apple juice in plastic cup with top 1 teaspoon Barley green or Solgar vitamin (green) powder, 1 tablespoon vegetable green protein powder, 1/2 teaspoon flaxseed oil or 1 teaspoon cod liver oil, 1 tablespoon choline, 1 teaspoon vitamin Ester C, 1/2 teaspoon honey or royal jelly, 1 tablespoon brewers yeast for B-Complex, 1 teaspoon kelp and wheat germ, shake well.*

*Fifth - Give first slot of vitamins labeled breakfast in vitamin box with vitamin juice above.*

*About 11AM - Sixth - Exercise (very important). Let her kick legs and arms 50 to 100 times. Then you pull arms and leg up, down, and all around at least 10 to 20 times as far as possible without pain. Also, deep breathing exercises (see attached).*

*Also, if possible let her roll around in kitchen in her wheelchair moving arms as well as legs. Give her water throughout the day. As much as possible but try to give at least 3 to 4 cups.*

*About 12:30Noon- Seventh - Lunch - feed her fruit and ensure nutritional drink or food. Give second slot in vitamin box labeled lunch with one glass of water.*

*Then give her lozenges - Calcium Citrate, 1 CoQ10, 1 B-12, proteolytic enzyme with SOD.*

*About 2:00 - In Between Lunch and Dinner - Give 1 or 2 Artho capsules and 2 MSM capsules with glass of water.*

*About 5:00 - Dinner - feed fruit/yogurt and food (depending upon what was eaten for lunch) and cup of water.*

*About 5:30 - After dinner transfer to restroom, rub joints with pain cream and transfer her to chair or to bed.*

*"And God gave us every herb bearing seed for our meat."     Genesis*

᭒᭒᭒᭒᭒᭒᭒᭒᭒᭒᭒᭒᭒

After practically living in the health food store for much of my lunch breaks, one of the ladies there gave me a phone number to a holistic practitioner since I had mentioned my mother's condition. She said this was a natural healing doctor who had treated an arthritic condition of one of her relatives and they had good results. She went on to say her condition was similar to Helen's in that she was confined to a wheelchair. Her body was gradually curving to the left and she had not walked for years. Hence, her muscles were contracted and her mind was starting to become clouded with irrational thoughts. The doctor she recommended lived in another state, but saw patients in Houston out of a hotel room about once a month. Being so desperate for healing, I finally was able to get Helen escorted by the city's handicap lift service. That was truly a miracle in itself considering how I telephoned time after time receiving numerous busy signals.

Once we were on our way to the holistic doctor, Helen complained about how far the doctor was. After arriving in the semi-luxurious hotel, we went up the elevator. Helen felt just as uncomfortable as I did, but never said too much. I pushed Helen to the corner of the room, filled out the paperwork and gave the doctor a list of medicinal herbs she was taking. The doctor was impressed and asked how did I know about these things, as I advised I had been reading about natural healing. After giving me some other natural healing products for my mother, she referred me to a colon clinic. She said all these problems stemmed from her toxic situation and once her system was cleansed, she would start the healing process.

This was no doubt the correct and profound analogy as I had concluded the same, but as it would prove most difficult to accomplish. Helen would never agree to have her colon cleansed. She has always been so head strong, and I barely coerced her into taking the vitamins and herbs let alone a colon cleansing. But I firmly believe if I had been able to acquire this treatment for Helen as well as diagnose any other possible digestive bacteria, we would have been able to immediately reverse her condition. I would later learn the bacteria called H. pylori affects the stomach lining as well as the duodenum, and causes ulcers. While some doctors treat the ulcer and never fully diagnose the cause of the problem which can be diagnosed and only monitored during the treatment process for complete healing via a breath test. H. Pylori bacterium can pass from mother to child, through dirty hands, feces, and just merely very contagious as it passes to another in close proximity of the affected person. Helen had been previously diagnosed and treated for ulcers and still had one, but had never taken a test such as a breath test to detect this bacteria as it mimics ulcer. Today, I strongly feel if the digestive track is healthy one may ultimately be able to live a disease free existence.

The holistic practitioner further prescribed an arthritic formula, a brain pill, and a digestive pill that included chlorophyll and acidophilus, a good bacteria which is depleted by the bad bacteria in the intestinal track.

As I continued to try and do what my mother allowed me to as far as a cleansing program, I included herbal bath products such as adding Epsom salt to bath water, as well as occasionally adding apple cider vinegar or other bath salts with chlorophyll for further pain relief. I bought bath brushes to help remove dead skin and open clogged pores as the skin not only protects, but it needs the ability to release some of the toxins from our bodies.

I further tried to correct our eating habits with a more balance regiment. For breakfast I continued to give her a scrambled egg as I had read eggs help balance the body, as you need some cholesterol. The good elements outweigh or offset any negative elements such as the yellow of an egg, which contains about two hundred fifteen milligrams of cholesterol. Even though I cooked it in olive oil along with a slice of whole grain flaxseed bread, I might have added fuel to the fire as our family's eating habits embodied years and years of a high fat and a cholesterol filled diet. After looking back on this situation, I now feel Helen's diet should not have been subjected to any additional cholesterol or animal fat, and I should have focused on a treatment to lower her cholesterol. As I feed her fresh fruit with yogurt or cottage cheese, and I

sometimes cooked lean meat in our vegetable stir-fry.  I eventually
started her on rice bread after I learned a lot of the starchy foods and
breads such as wheat, rye, barley, contain gluten and yeast.  Yeast can
cause mucous build up in your system.  I further learned that the gluten
in the bread could be linked to digestive problems such as irritable bowel
syndrome, as I took into consideration her previous stomach and
intestinal problems.  After much prayer and perseverance, Helen
continued to do well for the next three years.

      Considering how impaired my mother's condition appeared prior
to these dietary changes, seeing this dramatic change was nothing short
of a miracle.  Helen's progress was phenomenal, she came back to reality
as the hallucinations ceased, and could engage in daily conversations
with Rachel, her caregiver.

〰 〰 〰 〰 〰 〰 〰 〰 〰 〰 〰 〰

## Late 1999

      But one afternoon the unthinkable occurred once again, as
Rachel told me how Helen just snapped and seemed very irritable and
confused.  She eventually started talking to herself as though she was
seeing people, as she called out the names of various relatives from her
past.  I knew immediately Helen suffered a relapse.  Also little did I
know at the time, that hallucinations was a stroke symptom.  When
Rachel told me what happened, it seemed to be the most devastating day
of my life after three years of experiencing tremendous healing.  I still
relentlessly continued to try various cleansing herbal treatments, and
prayed and read the bible in between the hallucinating attacks that
rendered her sleepless for about three days at a time.  They were not very
often at first and she would always come back to a reasonably normal
state of mind, but they would eventually become more and more
frequent, almost weekly.  Unknown to me, this was not only a warning
sign or precursor to a massive stroke, but also I had started giving Helen
a brain formula with aspartame (an artificial sweetener) which has been
known to cause neurological disorders including brain cancer.  Although
she was not taking a large amount, I started to doubt everything I was

doing including my faith, and literally changed a lot of what I was doing right in an effort to correct this setback. I let this minor setback cause me to make even more mistakes. This was a warning sign but instead of correcting one error and possibly making one minor adjustment, I let this situation catapult into even more degradation as I felt like I went in the wrong direction. I felt as though I opened the door to an enemy in my life, and unfortunately one small often times unintentional compromise can lead to even larger eluding misconceptions. This was oddly enough the parallel disparity that had occurred throughout my own personal life.

☯ ☯ ☯ ☯ ☯ ☯ ☯ ☯ ☯ ☯ ☯ ☯

But as I continued to endeavor, I required assistance on the weekends and my brother, Fred, would sometimes help and my mother loved my brother's company. As they both loved to watch wrestling. Fred would bring over some videotapes while Helen would appear to have forgotten all about her ailments for that moment. She would always talk about the older wrestlers as though they were still there. " I saw that match, when I was at the coliseum last night, that's huh, that's, you know who I'm talking bout Fred", she exclaimed. As Fred would just reply, " Oh yea I know, look at that. Look, your missing it Helen", he replied. As he was able to get her mind back on track and they would laugh. I just watched and knew that her mind was continuing to deteriorate, as she had been recently diagnosed with Alzheimer's as well.

Fred and his wife, Marie, also graciously agreed to stay with Helen and my son Joseph, while I had my needed fibroid surgery. I had been delaying the surgery since Joseph's birth. They had grown with my pregnancy while recent stomach problems and additional weight gain, were no doubt deciding factors. Once I came home I felt so alone as I lay for two weeks unable to go downstairs. Helen on the other hand did pretty well as Rachel took care of her vitamin regiment while I was not able to go downstairs. Once I started to heal, I purchased Tae-Bo tapes in an effort to get myself back in shape. A few weeks after, I would then opt to have foot surgery. Hopping around on one-foot cleaning and transferring my mother, I could not heal correctly. But through it all, Helen was still my main concern.

As this situation started to wear on the family and everyone started to stay away. But I decided to continue researching and reading, as I once again returned to the quest for my mother's complete healing. Although Helen was doing better, she continued to exhibit bouts of memory loss symptoms as she mentioned her mother had the same problem and I continued to doubt myself. Then begun an extensive search into the cause and effect, with respect to our family history. Although my grandmother did take fairly good care of herself, she might have eaten a lot of excess sugar in her older years along with some hydrogenated oils, and cooked with thin aluminum pots. I noted the high sugar and metal toxicity, as Helen spoke of her mother eating lots of sweets such as peppermints, and cooking as well as eating from less than adequate pots and dishes. I felt proper nutrition and an adequate cleansing program might help deter this most devastating illness as she was diagnosed with Alzheimer's.

To try and combat the arthritis I further took Helen to a couple of specialist as someone had advised that the gold shots or injections in the affected area were helpful, but I could not locate a doctor that would still follow that arthritic treatment plan nor the natural chelation. Chelation is a relatively newer technology to help rid the body of heavy metals as well as arterial plague. But I did sometimes follow an oral chelated plan which included supplements such as alfalfa, sea kelp, garlic, grapefruit or apple pectin, coenzyme 10, 3000 to up to 5000 milligrams of Vitamin C with bioflavonoids, 400 up to 800 IU's of Vitamin E, chromium, selelium, L-Methionine, L-Cystiene, magnesium, potassium, and other chelated mineral supplements.

Then I finally was able to take to a facility that used whirlpool treatment for arthritic symptoms, but after examining Helen and seeing how contracted she appeared they said this treatment would not be advisable. As the futile search for my mother's treatment outside of what I was trying to do always ended up empty. It soon became painfully true that Helen would not be doing as well as she had been doing if I were not

supplementing her nutrition. I probably should have been happy with
how well she was doing, but as she was still having bouts of memory
losses along with the hallucinations, I continued my quest for her
healing.

✦ ✦ ✦ ✦ ✦ ✦ ✦ ✦ ✦ ✦ ✦ ✦ ✦ ✦ ✦

*Early 2000*

The medical supply company discontinued supplying her ensure,
as I had to start purchasing it again. I tried to continue to make sure I
keep it in the house, but sometimes she would run out. Also, trying to
maintain her nutrition while Helen's outbursts of memory loss and
confusion seem to become a weekly event lasting for at least three-day
intervals.

I further continued to seriously doubt myself and stop giving her
nutrients that I knew were beneficial such as parsley, other natural herbs
such as a little tumeric, natural brain nutrients such as DHA from sea
vegetables and cold water fish, while all the time relating all the
symptoms she was having to Alzheimer's disease. Never realizing how
much nutrition was in theses herbs and supplements including her
nutritional drinks. Further not realizing this condition could be
circulatory related, and could lead to other illnesses such as stroke.

Fred started to have problems with his car and on his job it
rendered him unable to continue helping out, I then asked my sisters if
they could resume helping by rotating one weekend per month.

Not long afterwards while my sister, Velma, was caring for
Helen, her speech started to slur as she loss conscious. She called me on
my mobil phone, "Nanette, there's something wrong with Helen. She
fainting and she's not talking right and oh no, now she throwing up". I
advised, "I will call 911 and meet you at the hospital". As this was one
of as many as four mini strokes in which Helen experienced while with
me, over the past six months. I could not figure out what was going on
with my mother, and so I simply attributed it to her previous condition of
diverticulitis a few years ago. As she would faint and vomit in the exact
same manner. When we would take her to the emergency room no one
told me what the problem entailed or even precautions, until a couple of

weeks before her massive stroke I took her to a different emergency room.  This doctor explained she might be having a mini stroke or what I later learned was called a TIA which was the warning sign that a massive stroke is nearing, he further advised that maybe I should start giving her a daily aspirin.  Considering I had taken her to other emergency room doctors and none had not mentioned or explained to me the issues surrounding a mini stroke or what to do.  I knew she had been previously diagnosed with diverticulitis and would experience fainting, rectal bleeding as well as vomiting with this condition.  Hence, I believed and thought for certain she was experiencing a relapse of her severe diverticulitis condition.  So I just increased her dosage of aloe vera along with a natural laxative and softeners.  I thought this was all related to the previously diagnosed condition, in so much as the attacks appeared exactly the same.  I did not have any previous knowledge or knew any of the symptoms of stroke or rather hardening of the arteries.

Both my sisters continued helping me for a few weekends, until Sophia advised her back was giving her problems and she would be unable to continue. Velma had another job on the weekend, which eventually took precedence.

As I continued my own research in light of the recent incidents while moving in the wrong direction, and literally unknown to me was a developing major problem. And in the weeks to come I would eventually not only question my actions but the doctors as well.  In that, was this last doctors' diagnosis just two weeks prior to her massive stroke enough time for me to alter what had been festering for years, and prevalent for 6 months.  Maybe the doctors could have possibly done a bit more, as they knew a mini stroke called a TIA as I would later learn was the precursor to a massive stroke, as I certainly did not.  Maybe as doctors they could have kept her in the hospital and performed more extensive tests considering how thick her blood was, maybe prescribed some medications to thin her blood?

For the next two weeks her right arm and leg continued to draw up, and I never thought about stroke nor was I aware of the symptoms.  I just continued to think it was the arthritis worsening along with symptoms of Alzheimer's disease and the diverticulitus. Hence, I merely continued to concentrate on the arthritic aspect of my mother's health, as it did not dawn on me that it could have been artery related symptoms such as a stroke or a heart attack from poor circulation because of hardening arteries. I continued to buy more books and read everything possible on health and nutrition, as I continued to accept the reality of being the primary caregiver for my mother. I read everything from pamphlets to magazines while concentrating on general nutrition, digestion problems, and arthritis. As I knew the information and knowledge was vast in these particular areas. I wish I could say we only tested a few herbs and vitamins but I cannot. My herbal research was quite in depth to say the least. To learn and enhance my knowledge even more, I decided to enroll in a distance education holistic college with a concentration in nutrition.

Also I recall slightly decreasing the amount of vitamin C and E Helen was taking, and increased her calcium intake for her arthritis. I further starting giving her an extra high protein drink for muscle and joint health, as her muscles appeared to be deteriorating.

As I would continue my learning quest, I decided to enroll in other more mainstream courses. I further decided I needed to return to one of my childhood aspirations, which meant going back to school and possibly concentrating in medicine. I always had the hope of one day becoming a doctor. It was not just a childhood dream, but I felt as though it was a calling in life from above.

✞ ✞ ♪♪♪♪♪♪♪♪♪♪♪♪♪♪ ✞ ✞

_Summer 2000_

Finally, I was able to return to a nearby local college, as the visiting skilled nurse's agency resumed sending a nurses assistant to feed and bath Helen at night.

My concentration was focused in pre-med and the first class I enrolled in was Anatomy and Physiology, as I had previously taken the course during my first years in college but lost interest and barely passed the course. But this time would be different, since my heart was back in line with my mind and I ended up receiving a course grade of an 'A'. But during my first semester the unexpected would occur. As my mother's caregiver, Rachel, arrived for the day she noticed Helen did not look right as she leaned to the side with her mouth a bit crooked. Rachel immediately went over to Helen as she lay in her recliner, as she tried talking to Helen. My mother's speech was slurred to the point that her spoken words were unrecognizable, and her right arm and leg was drawn up and virtually locked in place. I will never forget that hysterical call I received from Rachel, "Nanette something is wrong with Helen, she can't talk and her right side is all messed up". I advised her to call the ambulance as I met them at the hospital. As Helen lay quietly for over six hours in the emergency room as they ran test, they finally determined she had a massive stroke sometime during the night. The doctor encouraged me not to give her the medication to immediately reverse the stroke as they felt it would be to risky, and although I went along I have always felt they should have given or least offered her the medication upon her arrival. I would later learn this medication is given based on your weight and is sometimes called the clot busting medication. Some doctors further feel it can be given within the first 24 hours of a massive stroke. I was devastated by this most tragic incident and would have been even more distraught and possibly even given up, but as I had returned to college it served a bit of enlightenment. This course was to serve as a vehicle for a complete understanding of what happened to my mother.

Although this was a most tragic surprise, it was a blessing that I had enrolled in a class with an understanding instructor, Dr. Joseph Whitiker. As I advised him of the tragic event, Dr. Whitiker suggested that I fulfill a required five-page report by researching Cerebral Vascular Attack or more simply, a stroke. Thanks to Dr. Whitiker I was able to learn in detail about her most serious and delicate condition. I would later learn during my Anatomy & Physiology class that Helen had been having transient ischemic attacks (TIA's) or mini strokes for the prior six

months.  This was about the time I started back giving her arthritis
medication the doctor prescribed, which has also been identified to cause
plague to break a part and move through the arteries and possibly create
a blockage causing a stroke as well.

TIA's are a warning sign for an oncoming massive stroke and
caused my mother to have difficulty speaking, loose consciousness, start
to drool or vomit, and return back to normal within a few minutes.  As I
thought it was related to her existing diverticulitis, it turned out to be a
warning sign to a stroke or brain attack.  Not only can this condition be
brought on by a high fat and low fiber diet for most of one's life, I would
further learn some isolated substances are present in stroke patients such
as excessive amounts of glutamine, as well as high levels of the amino
acid creatine has been associated with strokes as well.

As Helen lay in the hospital for the next few days, I felt much
regret that I was totally unaware of that these transient attacks were a
warning sign that a full-blown stroke was nigh.  I recalled all her all
natural whole food supplements that probably kept her circulation up and
kept her a float before the onset of these attacks.  She ran out of garlic
and onions at times, and most importantly I had completely ran out of the
cayenne pepper capsules which are all good for circulation.  She also ran
out of some other herbs as well as I choose to discontinue some.

Only after Helen's condition climaxed did I gain a complete
understanding of hardening of the arteries, which can result in a stroke.
Types of stroke include thrombotic, embolic, or hemorrhagic
respectively.  Thrombosis is the major cause of stroke which entails a
blood clot build up (plague) inside the artery area, or embolus which are
moving blood clot deposits that break off and enter the intricate ranging
proportion arterial system.  Blood clots can entail bad cholesterol
attaching itself to calcium that can involve vitamin K as well as a protein
called fibrinogen attaching to platelets to form a clot, which is the body's
normal response to a damaged artery.  The bad cholesterol cannot be
absorbed by the body properly as it can move in the arterial system or
buildup sticking platelets (thick blood) creating narrowing and ultimately
blockages in the arterial circulatory system. Lastly a hemorrhage entails

bleeding in or around the brain and normally associated with hypertension due to drug or alcohol use and symptoms can be as small as a minor headache.

Although giving my mother some vitamins such as antioxidants C and E protect the body against the effects of some destructive free radical damage including pollution, bad water, there is still some other damage to the arteries that accumulate overtime. Other free radical damage can come from varying sources. Eating bad food such as foods high in saturated fats, fried in certain vegetable oils, oils that solidify at room temperature such as lard, palm, and coconut oils, meat products, hydrogenated oils, birth control pills, and smoking just to mention some of the risk factors.

After the initial attack oxygen is inhibited to the brain cells, and cells die creating extensive damage but the damage can be reversed since the medical community has made profound strides by the discovery of clot busting drugs. If the attack does not result in death drugs can be administered within hours if one seeks immediate medical attention, but this was something Helen was not given. As she sat in the ER over six hours without any treatment, I later found out how thick Helen's blood was at the time. I feel the drug should have been administered as her normal course of treatment. This drug would have given her an opportunity to regain her normal faculties as she could not speak at all for awhile and when she did eventually speak, she never regained her normal speaking ability. As I feel patients should have the opportunity to be administered this drug up to twenty-four hours of a stroke, as the risk in most cases is worth the possibility of living life without being able to communicate. As her speech tried to emerge after a couple of days of treatment with Heparin, but only resulted in one or two understandable utterances. She would never again be able to tell me if she was hurting, hungry, or any vital information that may be crucial for me to care for her. Once taken off the Heparin, she would further continue start having repeated TIA's again, the precursor, and indication to me that another eventual massive stroke could occur.

Arterial blockage can occur in an artery directly associated with the heart resulting in a heart attack, or an artery associated with the brain creating a brain attack or stroke. Brian attack refers to thrombotic or embolic strokes, which occur primarily due to insufficient blood flow to the brain due to a blockage, or a hemorrhagic stroke refers to bleeding in the brain from a blood vessel. As the normal blood flow stops, vital nutrients as well as oxygen supplies also cease and just like the TIA's my mother was experiencing, this was one of the major warning signs of a massive or full-blown stroke was nigh. Sadly, statistics suggest most people remain unaware of this most vital information, and quite tragically choose to ignore these signs or symptoms. Symptoms such as irritability, confusion, weakness, dizziness, difficulty walking, numbness, loss of consciousness, nausea, vomiting, difficulty speaking, pain in one part of the body or maybe a routine headache. Most people have an unrealistic sense of immortality and do not realize the grave consequences of not heeding the most significant warning signs. We can and must pay close attention to our bodies and respond appropriately and timely or we will receive the most devastating consequences. I have further learned there are arterial scans that can be done to detect artery blockage or hardening of the arteries. Most can be surgically removed if detected in time.

I would later learn a lot more. As we age, it is inevitable that our arteries will become less pliable or weak due to the hardening. Hence, all persons should invest in a scan of the head or neck, heart or abdominal, as well as the leg arteries. This scan should not be taken lightly and if blockage or build up is detected, it followed up on immediately and treated as this may be difference in you having a stroke or heart attack or rather living or dying. I other words, early detection can not only prevent these devastated situations, but can also save your life.

Additionally, we need dietary changes to circumvent this circulatory problem. To keep blood flowing properly through the arteries, the bad cholesterol (LDL's), are primarily derived from consuming high saturated fat food and hydrogenated oil which can be prevented or decreased by proper diet. The good cholesterol (HDL's) must be higher or increased to help avoid heart attacks and stroke. Foods rich in monounsaturated fats such as certain nuts and cooking oils can lower cholesterol. *More specifically natural nut butters or nuts such as pecans, almonds, cashews and macadamia are considered good fats that help lower cholesterol.* Oils such as olive, high heat safflower, and. macadamia oil are high in monounsaturated fat and can lower cholesterol. Additionally even if these oils are used with high heat such as frying or baking, they may not become toxic to the body. As heating high polyunsaturated oils releases some substances that has been known to change the oils chemical composition, which can result in toxicity to the body. Basically good oils that are high in polyunsaturated fats should not be heated such as cold pressed omega 3 oils found in flaxseed, which is an essential oil for tissue health and regeneration.

Omega 3 are also found in some fish such as salmon, tuna, herring, trout, and mackerel. Along with consuming adequate antioxidants, a good absorbable glocosamine and chondroitin supplement, magnesium along with some other nutritional supplements. Also most important are high fiber foods such as natural whole grains, seeds, nuts, and whole grain soy products, and possibly some blood thinners (aspirin) as well as natural artery chelation (cleansers) could help break up the artery deposits. I later found as a preventative measure Helen should have started taking a daily aspirin in her forties in addition to proper dietary habits, which all could have helped alleviate excess coagulate in her blood. But further recent studies are continuing to find that aspirin, because of the circulatory benefits may help prevent other sicknesses and disease such as Alzheimer's.

I was just devastated as I sat in her hospital room every evening after work and weekends lining her room with what I called good oxygenated plants, while trying to figure out the why's, yet trying to remain hopeful she would fully recover from this massive stroke. Inquiring about her condition, as her regular doctor was not involved, because I had to take her to the nearest hospital and he was not affiliated with hospital. The resident doctor at the hospital wanted to immediately put a feeding tube in my mother's stomach, but as my brother Fred I was hesitant, the doctor agreed to evaluate her swallowing. Before the test was returned, they put the tube down her throat to feed her, where it was kept until she entered the rehab center. The doctor advised the hospital's physical therapy unit would not be able to provide her with the level of rehabilitation she needed. He further advised she would be going to less vigorous rehabilitation center as they felt she was not responsive enough. One of the hospital therapists that were working with Helen advised she was during well and hoped she would be accepted into the hospital's rehabilitation unit. I felt the same way and was deeply saddened at this decision, as I knew she heard and understood everything I said. I would make the following request to my mother just as the therapist, "Helen kick your leg, kick your leg Helen". I would touch her leg slightly helping her along then she would begin to respond with a kick. She probably would have did a lot better and her condition would not have regressed into even more strokes, and further unresponsiveness if she had been allowed that chance. In an effort to do anything I possibly could I brought vases full of ivy, philodendron, and an aloe vera plant, in order to help facilitate and increase the level of oxygen in her hospital room. I knew these plants help supply oxygen as she needed all the help she could get for her healing. My coworkers had also sent a wonderful plant. It was a beautiful ivy that I still kept in her room next to her bed even after she returned home.

After they transferred Helen into the rehab center I watched Helen's condition closely visiting her daily, traveling over fifteen miles there and back as I sometimes visited her on my lunch breaks and throughout the day. They finally let me start to feed her pureed foods only after her feeding tube accidentally came out of her nose, the nurses tried to put it back and nearly took all her breathe away. I watched the incident as they attempted to slide the tube down, which ended up being shoved down the throat. As I watched and cringed in pure freight with my hands quenching my face, until I finally requested them to leave her alone. The following day after a swallowing test, they decided she could eat pureed foods. I further requested additional ensure supplements.

Her stay at the rehabilitation center did not go well, as I had to plead with them to do any level of therapy. They complained she was uncooperative but they never talked or tried some level of reasonable interaction, as she desired for you to communicate with her as well as she was in pain. I felt their level of expertise was not up to par. I asked the doctor to put her back on her arthritic medication and maybe it would help her cooperate while easing the pain. I recall not long after that medication she had yet another TIA, as I did not know what caused the stroke the doctor put her on a low dosage blood pressure pill and I asked him to discontinue the arthritis medication. I continued to search for more help but to no avail, as other rehabs I contacted would not accept her. I knew it was a no win situation, as her insurance would probably not allow the continued rehab. So I sat filled with dismay, as they discontinued the little therapy they were providing. Then I started to request for her immediate release.

I knew Rachel, her daily caregiver, could do more for her on a daily basis than they were willing to give in the rehab. Although Helen still could not talk, from the first day home Rachel started to help Helen by kicking her legs, trying to lift her arms, and moving her neck from side to side. Rachel knew just as I that exercise kept Helen going, and this was no doubt anything less than a true call from heaven above as Rachel was truly God sent. Although it did not seem like very much exercise to the average person, it was actually saving my mother's life. Helen was very responsive to conversation. Although her words were not very understandable we did grasp a few words such as yes and no, but some nurses who were familiar with stroke victims understood her every word. The only other major drawbacks from this massive stroke was not having the ability to feed herself as well as eat regular foods. As her ability to swallow was compromised, we were required to give her thickened pureed foods.

Although she maintained her ability to chew, we basically did not feed her any solid foods. I decided to change her diet once again, I decided to take *her off the eggs yolks and all meat products* after the research paper I did in class on stroke. As her blood was thick and circulation poor, I discontinued any foods that might contribute to the already bad situation. Then I started mixing her egg substitute with 1/4cup brown rice milk, and sometimes added soy lecithin granules. Although I stopped a lot of the herbs such as kelp, and alfalfa as well as spirulina as I thought too much vitamin k might not be helping her current problem. I did continue mixing some herbs such as garlic, onion, ginger, and a few other culinary spices. In an attempt to reverse this condition, her diet contained primarily pureed vegetarian food. I tried giving her more whole grains such as barley, wheat, and rye but discontinued due to her possible gluten sensitivity and previous bowel problems, and I just added pureed nuts. Her diet mostly contained fresh purred lentils, some other bean combination such as black bean and kidney with pureed corn and quinoa for her complete protein. Also I included lots of vegetables and herbal seasonings. I changed the her information on the refrigerator to read as follows:

*Helen's Tasks*

*About 8:00AM - First task before cleaning up - 1 cup of water. Next mix ½ banana or pureed fruit with 2 capsules magnesium/potassium/bromelin combination, 1 magnesium orotate, 2 cap MSM/glucosamine/ascorbyl palmitate combination, and 1/4 teaspoon apple pectin for colon health as needed.*

*Please note: Give one glass of water before pureed fruit, as water might wash away the nutrients. Always give her a few sips of water with meals, but basically give full cups in between her meals.*

*Second task - Clean-up/Bathe with natural bath wash (aloe vera & antioxidants) and put lotion all over body and olive oil mixture (tea tree oil, vitamin E, lavender, wild yam) on joints and back as the oil helps arthritis and joint stiffness as well as the dry skin areas. About 9:00 - Third - Fix Breakfast - please use ½ cup rice or soy milk, 1 egg white with 1/3 cup egg substitute with add all seasonings on turntable on countertop. Also note plenty of fenugreek, rosemary, thyme, garlic and onion powder. After egg has cooled a bit grind pills, 1 Plavix and ½ Aspirin, ½ blood pressure pill with one part of egg substitute, let her eat that portion first, than pureed the rest of the egg, four fig/apple or raspberry cookies, and ½ cup of tea.*

*Note: As the doctor prescribe her pills in 30-day intervals; let me know when low so I can call for refills. As her pressure remains almost normal (averaged 120/60) I give her ½ dosage.*

*About 11 AM - Forth - Exercise (very important). Moving limbs and holding the position until arms/legs relax, then move limb further without force allowing her to relax again. Also if possible try to get her sit-up on bed or sit her up in recliner for 2 to 3 hours.*

*Give her water throughout the day.  As much as possible but try to give at least 3 to 4 cups.*

*Give vitamin mixture. The fresh juice (greens, carrots, celery, beets, apples, mango) with 1 teaspoon powdered barley, ½ capsule  nacinamide, 1/4 teaspoon vitamin (ester) C, 1 teaspoon honey or royal jelly, 1 capsule of B-complex with taurine, 1 capsule pycnogenol or 1 grape seed capsule for additional vitamin C and E, 1 capsule CoQ10 with lecithin, 500mg magnesium orotate, 250mg L-methionine, 1000mcg to 5000mcg of B12 lozenge, maitake D fraction with beta glucans to boost immune system, one 250 to 500mg brain nutrition capsule (acetyl-carnitine, ginkgo with phosphatidal serine and bilberry), anti-aging capsule (alpha lipoic acid, ascorbyl palmitate non acidic vitamin C) at least twice a week, and shake well.*

*Please note if she does not want vitamin mixture try to give as much as possible before lunch.*

*About 12:30 - Lunch – Additionally to help lower cholesterol: Pureed beans/rice/corn/pureed macadamia nut butter and fruit, 2 capsules magnesium, 1 capsule IP-6 hexanicotinate a form of flush free niacin cholesterol lowering herbal capsule for circulation, and/or vegetarian nutritional drink.*

*About 2:00 - Before leaving change her and rub joints with pain cream and put her in bed.*

*About 5:00 - Dinner - Pureed food (depending upon what was eaten for lunch) and cup of water and/or night vitamins if unable to sleep (100mg melatonin, passion flower with magnesium, garlic, and hawthorn berries, etc).*

Additional Nutritional Notes:

I mixed her vitamins daily for whomever cared for Helen during the week. I also made Helen a natural lotion for the face and body.  It includes olive oil, aloe vera, tea tree oil to fight bacteria, lavender oil to help relax her, vitamin E which is even excellent alone as a nighttime moisturizer.  The mixture is also good for hair moisturizing, and the joints for more mobility.  Also, sometimes I add wild yam moisturizer since it is excellent for balancing hormones as I use it as well.  As I concentrate on the underarm, chest, and stomach areas for absorption.  I also use a morning cream and beta glucan that helps to clean the face pores of dirt and help destroy the unwanted toxins.  Beta glucan can be derived from various sources.  For my face cream it is derived oats, and for my nutritional supplement it is derived from maitake mushrooms.  It is known for helping to boost the immune system and destroy foreign substances such as viruses, bacteria, tumor cells, and heavy metal toxins.

I felt trying everything in its natural state would proof to be a healthier lifestyle.  We did not even eat any processed or smoked foods as the probability increases for lost of nutritional value, and the food may even gain toxins from the process.  As most of the additives to our food such as colors, artificial flavors, and preservatives have been tested and produced cancer in laboratory animals.  Hence, I tried to consciously avoid all unnatural forms of food keeping a log of my findings while trying to maintain a strict regiment and make adjustments.

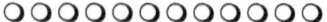

About two weeks after Helen's hospital visit, she had another TIA. I tried desperately to have her medication changed. Until her primary care physician advised us to bring her into the hospital for observation. She had developed an infection in her legs, from what the doctor said was bruises. I feared we might have hit her legs on the wheelchair during transferring her from the bed. But she was also dehydrated. Finally after a few weeks, she came home only to go back within in few short weeks.

Again she had another TIA, but I contacted a cardiologist I met on the elevator from her previous hospital stay. He said she was dehydrated again, and recommended she take the 80 mg aspirin only each day instead of the current medication. I decided to give her the 80 mg aspirin daily, as well as increase her water intake. I also started mixing at least 1/4 to 1/2 cup of water with all her food and giving her a full twelve-ounce tumbler of water in the morning, afternoon, and at night for the dehydration. I further felt due to her age as well as the fact she continued to have the TIA's that a Helen needed to continue her current medication, because I knew Helen could not at her age handle another full-blown stroke. Hence, she was in the hospital once again from another mini-stroke or TIA. The neurologist finally ran a few tests and continued the 75mg tablet of plavix an anti-platelet drug, and the 80mg aspirin daily as I continued to give the arthritic medication for her pain as well.

After Helen's third hospital visit, Rachel, her caregiver who had found another job because of Helen's frequent hospital stays and was only working half days, left for good. Another caregiver was taking care of Helen during the day. I had changed agencies and know that it did not help matters any, but they had problems sending a backup if Rachel needed to be off. Also, the company did not pay if the patient was in the hospital. Although I totally understood, at times I would feel so alone after Rachel left us. She was the only person I could depend on for my mother's care. Then our family friend, Charlene, who came into our lives few years after Daddy's death would once again try to help, as she would eventually end up in the hospital for a TIA herself. She advised me that her doctor diagnosed her with a tumor behind her eye as her vision became fuzzy. As she refused to have surgery, I advised Charlene to do something about her condition as I advised it might be Cushing's because of her extensive cortisol based arthritis treatment. I continued to talk with her occasionally, trying to help her change her diet and visit the health food store with me. I also would try to give her some information that would help her, as she had high blood pressure and diabetes as well. One afternoon as she visited I gave her a couple of garlic tabs and cayenne pepper capsules for her circulation, also some culinary herbs with quinoa, split peas, and corn. I further gave her some other vitamins and herbs I gave Helen. She later advised that night she was painless, and further advised I was doing good things for Helen. I also continued to research her condition and advise her of some medicinal precautions.

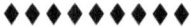

As I continued to need help with Helen after her stroke, a pleasant and unexpected change occurred. My brother Charles, who had remained in the background as far as my mother's care, started to occasionally assist me with Helen's care. Although Charles always called to check on her and visited as often as he could, he stayed his distance mainly because I did not like his drinking sometimes. I know from my father's side drinking was very prevalent, as they drank to ease the pain and it no doubt passed down to us. As I finally received nothing short of a miracle when I conquered my drinking problem before my son was born, as I continued to pray daily for this curse to be broken. Finally despite my continued nagging, Charles helped me faithfully as he caught the bus over to my house and stayed overnight for a few days at a time, as I would have to pick him up and drop him off at the bus stop. Considering Charles eventually took a bout of illness himself, I had to go back and forth using my lunch breaks, as the caregiver would sometimes not arrive as planned. The agency that provided daytime care for Helen hired a lady that was unable to arrive on time. I ended up having to wait for her as I found she would not arrive at my house until sometimes

midmorning. She cared for her ailing mother as well who had blood
clots, and asked me to write down foods I eat and give to Helen. I gladly
wrote down almost two pages of foods to avoid such as all white flour
products including bread, cookies and pastries as well as beef, pork, and
a lot cooked foods. I further wrote down all the herbs I used and advised
her to eat more fresh vegetables and fruit, and cooked foods should
include mostly brown rice, and beans such as soy or black beans, etc.
Although I probably will never know if she actually followed my list, I
do know God allows certain people to touch our lives for a reason. I
would only hope that somehow in my life I have helped someone and it
was not all in vane.

Considering Helen could not be left alone all morning, I finally
had to switch to yet another agency as they immediately sent another
caregiver, but she would soon leave. I was once again having to change
and feed Helen before work. Although this agency was more reliable
and would send replacement caregivers as needed, I would still have to
sometimes prepare her breakfast as well as her lunch. I continued to
prepare her vitamin mixture and mostly cooked her breakfast since they
sometimes had to send different caregivers.

As I recalled before Rachel came to us how I prayed to God
would send a good person to help care for my mother, and he did. I
knew that God had not left me, as the agency would finally hire a second
lady full time to care for my mother. As I hoped everything would work
I just continued to read my bible as often as possible, and if I am unable
to read as I desire I still read the following verses almost daily. As these
verses give me the strength to continue and make me feel blessed that
God has chosen me to help care for a person in need, and who happens to
be my mother. As I would read the book of Saint John chapter eleven,
verses forty-three through forty-four, "And when he had thus spoken,
he cried out in a loud voice, *Lazarus, come forth. And he that was dead came
forth, bound hand and foot with grave clothes and his face was bound about
with a napkin. Jesus saith unto them, Loose him, and let him go.*" I no doubt
feel Jesus was the reason why I survived all my many mistakes, as well
as my mother surviving so many ailments and disease. And although

neither one of us is what one would consider perfect, my mother is here with me and I with her. I knew it was nothing short of a miracle for the both of us.

As my life was what one might call rather hectic I decided to work part time, but everything seemed to remain about the same except my income. Although insurance covered her monthly supplies I would constantly have to keep involved to obtain the doctors information and signatures to keep slim list of supplies. As I always run out of the wipes, pads, and the diapers every now and then. But I would eventually go back to work full-time after becoming financially burdened.

She also would still sometimes have skin breakdowns and the nurse provided daily take care of her foot, but as they finally finished the antibiotic her body was so imbalanced. I thought I would loose her as they managed to acquire an over three-inch hole in her foot. I started to give her Miatake 'D' Fraction, a mushroom extract to help boost her immune system. I further started using a liquid silver crème. Finally, she started back resting through the night as she began to heal. I began feeling much better about her condition and this allowed me to return back to work full time with ease.

In the meantime I further had to still try to and raise a son, which proved to be a challenge considering he was now a teenager. But as he was still very understanding and dedicated to his studies, I feel very fortunate. But during this most trying time following Helen's stroke, I started to neglect my health as I stopped exercising, started eating incorrectly, and began to feel tired and run down as I gained twenty-five pounds.

One of my coworkers noticed what was once a small knot and unnoticeable. Dina exclaimed, "Nette, what's that on your neck. It looks like a knot". I advised that it had been there since my first car accident over eighteen years ago, but it was so small I could barely see it. I knew I had to do something as I had gained over twenty-five pounds over the last six months, and this small knot had gotten noticeably larger. Only a few months later I developed another small lump in my pelvic area and chest area. My doctor had been trying to get me back unto the office since last year, because my pap smear was slightly abnormal and he wanted to re-test. As I procrastinated for months, I knew I needed to try and reverse these effects. I had been through this weight gain and losing weight regimen too many times for a total loss of more than one hundred and sixty pounds overtime. It was getting harder with age and I could not believe once again this five foot tall person was one hundred and sixty five pounds.

The very first time I became overweight was while pregnant with my son, Joseph. While the baby averages between seven to eight pounds, doctors only allow about twenty pounds for the fluid. At 5 feet tall I went from about 115 pounds to 170 pounds in nine months. I was miserable, as I could not even lie in the bed due to having difficulty breathing. That was why I spent my pregnancy lying on the couch with my feet up, and upper body in an upright sitting position. And within a couple of years I went down to a size eight only to return to an overweight situation in the following two years. At 165 pounds once again at the age of thirty-one I looked about ten years older. As I attempted my weight loss once again I gained assistance from a couple of coworkers. I went to the spa daily and Cynthia, a coworker, who became my exercise buddy. Another coworker, Bobbie, let me borrow a book she purchased on fat burners. As I learned I began to eat more of the _fat burner foods_ such as citrus fruits and vegetables.

ꔹ ꧁ ꧁ ꧁ ꧁ ꔹ

Nutritional Notes:
Fruits and vegetables not only contain essential vitamins, but some of these foods contain pectin which helps remove toxins such as heavy metals from your body as they metabolize and move the fat out of our bodies. This includes fruits such as apples and grapefruit. Also oranges, lemons, and limes are good cleansers. Some other fruits high in vitamin C as well as E include kiwi and strawberries.
Melons are also great fat burners such as cantaloupe, watermelon, and I later learned watermelon is best if eaten first, alone, or with small meals, as most fresh fruits digest quickly. Fruits if eaten after a large meal can literally sit in your stomach and rot creating a toxic environment. But watermelon can be essential to a weight loss program, and cantaloupe can be added to a daily regiment as well.
I also eat fat burner vegetables such as broccoli, beets, celery, carrots, cauliflower, and sometimes I include other fat burners such as tomatoes and cucumbers. Cauliflower, broccoli, brussel sprouts, kale, and cabbage are considered cruciferous vegetables, which are excellent for colon health and even help, fight colon cancer. Cauliflower is further considered a brain nutrient as it contains choline, an essential brain nutrient. You can also sometimes determine what a vegetable is good for

by how it looks, as cauliflower looks like a brain and beets are red and good for the blood. Additionally as a child I had previously learned from Mrs. Matthew's, a teacher and family friend, that a tablespoon of apple cider vinegar along with a glass of water burned fat. Not only is it a good fat burner, but apple cider vinegar is also a good for blood pressure and cholesterol. I try to drink this occasionally as a tea with honey. Honey is also filled with nutrients that are vital to the body as well as enzymes. As we age our enzymes decrease and I try to take enzymes as often as possible to help digest food, and they are further essential to heal other health conditions and disease.

ᛒ ᗰᗰ ᗰᗰ ᗰᗰ ᗰᗰ ᛒ

I learned that enzymes might protect from brain diseases such as Alzheimer's to helping my fibroid cyst, a condition that I developed while pregnant with Joseph.

One year before Helen stop walking, I recalled how I lost forty-five pounds. I went from one hundred and sixty-five pounds to one hundred and twenty-pounds, I then decided to reward myself by entering a beauty contest. As salesperson had mentioned to me that a Miss Petite Beauty Pageant was registering for contestants. In preparation for the pageant in Dallas, I enrolled in a preparation class. A former beauty pageant contest winner offered it, and she demonstrated walking, facial expressions, and other techniques. Although I felt I never really mastered it, I did end up number seventeen in the competition. I modeled a lovely Lillie Ruben gown, but it was not enough to win. A lady from the Woodlands won the contest as her walk, facial expressions, and weight was a perfect one hundred and ten pounds and she deserved to win. But I enjoyed the contest experience as I made it into a vacation taking a plane there, while my sisters rented a van and brought my son and their kids as well. As we returned from the contest in Dallas, I recall that day how Helen just sat and barely talked, as she stated her desire to have joined us in Dallas. Little did I know her health was taking a downward turn never quite realizing the magnitude, or impact of her illness. Seeing how I tried to start her on vitamin C ascorbic acid and calcium carbonate to give her energy and combat the arthritis, it just made her worst. Considering that both forms of the supplements were not very good for the body, nor were they very absorbable forms as I later learned and would discontinue use only after a few weeks.

But the next time I would gain weight, it would not be as bad.  About year after we moved into the new house I gradually went back up to one hundred and forty pounds.  Enjoying the new house and just getting cozy with an entire bag of my vinegar and sea salt flavored potato chips, was definitely not helping my weight situation.  As I began to return to the exercise spa for the second time almost daily on my lunch breaks, I created a weekly reminder in my calendar:  The subject was *"Fruit Fast"*, it stated, *"Eat Fruits/Vegetables All Day"*, and the reminder started on Thursday at 7:30 a.m. and ended on Friday at 4:00 p.m.  The reminder further stated, *"If you have to eat food, eat ONLY high* **PROTEIN** *and fiber with low fat and low carb food and* ***EXERCISE*** *at lunch to keep a healthy heart rate, mind, and whole body"*.

Considering I took the time to make this weekly reminder while bolding the words like protein and exercise, one would think I would never have been overweight again, wrong.  Although I must admit it did help me, as I continued to strive for perfection.  I still needed a set plan of what foods to eat.  Then I went back on a diet program as I had several diets from my sisters and friends.  Most of which I had good results, but as I continued to try to eat right I created my own regular daily diet plan and it worked pretty well.  Because I found you must have a plan for your daily diet, just like any other task or job in your life.  If you do not have a plan, you will eat anything and everything.  I further had to keep the plan with me, as I made a small copy and used a hole-punch to add it to the front of my folio planner.  I further had to cut out a clear sheet protector cover to keep it in good condition.  I use it almost on a weekly basis, and carry my planner with me daily as I finally realized that healthy living is a lifestyle.

꜀ ᨬ ᨬ ᨬ ᨬ ꜀

Nutritional Notes:

When I am not on this diet I try to still eat high protein such as turkey, chicken, or vegetable protein and no more than 2 to 4 ounces per meal.  But more over high fiber foods such as complex carbohydrates, which assist in maintaining healthy weight as well as assist in weight loss.  High fiber foods include fruits, vegetables, whole grain breads, and cereals such as kashi.  Also I sometimes include split peas with whole grains such as quinoa as well as seeds and natural nuts (no additives).

In this diet I attempted to reflect a more realistic weight loss of no more than three to five pounds per week.  I further included tea, herbal seasonings, meat alternatives, and included only coldwater fish, which is most nutritious and helps lower your cholesterol.  Also I sometimes added a half-cup of coffee or green tea for breakfast to increase the metabolism or rather fat burning process, but then I discovered some delicious dark chocolate bars without any carbohydrates. I also found some wonderful protein bars, which have low to no carbohydrates and no hydrogenated oils. The chocolate bars have zero net carbohydrates and chocolate is considered a powerful antioxidant with polyphenols that can be just as good for the heart as red wine. I further added some options such as alfalfa sprouts and mix with vegetables, seasonings such as lemon juice and boca burgers, a meat substitute, together as a delicious salad as it read as follows:

*LOOSE THREE TO FIVE POUNDS IN FOUR DAYS*

*YOU WILL HAVE THE FOLLOWING BREAKFAST FOR FOUR DAYS WHICH INCLUDES AT LEAST <u>ONE CUP OR MORE OF TEA</u> CHOICES SUCH AS: RED or GREEN TEA and/or YOGI BRAND BRAIN TEA FORMULA WITH HERBS SUCH AS GINGKO TEA,LEMONGRASS,BACOPA and CELESTIAL SEASONINGS DETOX TEA (MILK THISTLE, DANDELION, RED CLOVER, ECHINACE) ALONG GARCINIA TEA AND ONE HALF GRAPEFRUIT.*
*USE ONLY LEMON JUICE AND/OR APPLE CIDER VINEGAR, AND A LITTLE OLIVE OIL FOR SEASONING. OTHER SEASONING ALLOWED: SEA SALT, THYME, OREGANO, ONION, GARLIC, FENNEL, CAYENNE PEPPER, PARSLEY, FENUGREEK, GROUND FLAX SEEDS, SUNFLOWER SEEDS, SESAME SEEDS, DILL WEED. SOME OTHER HERBS OR SEASONINGS ACCEPTABLE: SUCH AS KELP GRANULES, ROSEMARY, AND CUMMIN, IF YOU LIKE YOU CAN.DRINK TEA DURING THE DAY. TEAS SUCH AS RED CLOVER, UVA URSI, MILK THISLE, ORANGE-GINGER, & IF DRINKING DIET TEA PLEASE USE AS DIRECTED ONLY. PLEASE NOTE: YOU CAN INCLUDE OTHER INGREDIENTS WITH YOUR SALAD SUCH AS RED ONIONS, RADISHES, AND CUCUMBERS AS THEY ARE ALL CONSIDERED FAT BURNERS AS WELL.*

<u>*DAY ONE*</u>      LUNCH: 1 OR 2 HARD BOILED EGG WHITES, ASPARAGUS, 1/2 GRAPEFRUIT
DINNER: BROILED STEAK OR MEAT EQUIVALENT (i.e. VEGGIE BURGER)
WITH MUSHROOMS SALAD - FRESH MIXED GREENS AND/OR
ALFALFA SPROUTS, FRESH TOMATOES, AN APPLE

<u>*DAY TWO*</u>      LUNCH: SALAD -FRESH SQUASH, FRESH CAULIFLOWER, FRESH ASPARAGUS,
APPLESAUCE OR AN APPLE
DINNER: FISH (TUNA, SALMON, TROUT, OR COD) or MEAT SUBSTITUTE
SALAD - MIXED GREENS AND/OR ALFALFA SPROUTS, TOMATOES

<u>*DAY THREE*</u>      LUNCH: MEAT EQUIVALENT: VEGGIE BURGER OR PROTEIN SUBSTITUTE
SALAD - FRESH CELERY AND MIXED GREENS AND AN APPLE
DINNER: BROILED CHICKEN AND SHITAKE MUSHROOMS, STEWED TOMATOES,
SMALLGLASS PRUNE JUICE

<u>*DAY FOUR*</u>      LUNCH: 1or 2 COOKED EGG WHITES, ASPARAGUS, SMALL GLASS TOMATO JUICE
DINNER: BROILED STEAK OR MEAT EQUIVALENT WITH SHITAKE MUSHROOMS,
MIXED GREENS, TOMATO, AND FRESH PINEAPPLE

*NOTE:IF YOU WOULD LIKE TO EAT THE EGG YOLK, EAT NO MORE THAN ¼ OF THE HARD BOILED YOLK FOR ADDITONAL NUTRITION. HENCE TRY TO EAT ALL THINGS IN NORMAL SIZE PROPORTIONS. ALSO WHEN YOU ARE NOT ON THEFOUR DAY DIET ALWAYS CONTINUE TO EAT RRIGHT AND INCLUDE LOTS OF VEGGIE'S,*
*FRUITS. ALSO ALWAYS INCLUDEA GOOD WHOLE FOOD MULTIPLE VITAMIN DAILY AND "MAY GOD RICHLY BLESS YOU."*
Additional Nutritional Notes:
Also I found too many non-complex carbohydrates help stimulate the production of fat as they contain yeast and virtually no fiber. So as our diet should contain at least 20 percent of carb's, and those carbohydrates can include your fruit, vegetables, and whole grains, as all are high in fiber. A high fiber diet can promote weight loss. Some high fiber kashi cereals can contain up to eight or

more grams of fiber per cup. You can also include additional rice bran, which is very high in fiber, which can contain up to 19 grams per half-cup. Rice bran not only provides high fiber but also can contribute to lowering your bad cholesterol. Additionally about 30 grams of fiber per day is recommended. Too much cooked food including white breads and pasties are low in fiber and filled with sugar or rather simple carbohydrates. By taking out most of the fiber from whole grain, we loose most of our most needed nutrition of whole grain or complex carbohydrates and then substitute it with empty simple carbohydrates. The fiber or germ has been removed in white flour products. White flour has been altered just as white sugar, removing all the vital substances to aid in a healthy lifestyle. Leaving most of us overweight, as I ate too much cooked foods such as white bread, white sugar, and animal fat, and not enough fresh fruits and vegetables. Eating too much cooked and low-fiber foods literally stops the body up, and cannot be digested as normal. This obstructs body fluidity causing fat buildup, mucus, and congestion. To help solve this problem I try to eat more fruits and vegetables as they are filled with nutrients and digestible enzymes that the body needs, and are vital to maintain optimum health. I try to eat at least a half of grapefruit in the morning along with my herbal teas, such as ginkgo, in between my scheduled regimented diets.

As I had wonderful results about four years ago from this diet of eating fresh organic fruits in the morning especially grapefruit along with apples as they help remove toxins. Further adding mostly fresh organic vegetables such as red onions and leafy green salad mix. Onions may be useful in lowering cholesterol and decreasing tumor growths. I tried to create a diet for myself to reflect these foods. After realizing fresh fruits and vegetables are filled with digestive enzymes and undigested food turns into fat, I tried to eat fresh as often as possible.

ᔕᔕᔕᔕᔕᔕᔕᔕᔕᔕᔕᔕᔕᔕᔕᔕᔕᔕᔕ

## Late 2000

As I returned to the doctor the knot on my neck had gotten smaller and the pelvic lump had completely disappeared as I had loss about twenty pounds. As we tested the lump on my neck as well as repeat the pap, everything was returned negative. After I received that good news I started to cheat a little. On the off days of my diet I sometimes eat a couple of slices of my son's pizza, although I do try to put additional fresh vegetables including red onions while sprinkling a enzyme capsule, to enhance my digestion and nutrition content. I further tried to throw away most of the thick crust. Anytime I eat flour products with yeast such as tortilla's, white bread, or other none whole grain products my system goes into what I call shut down and I just gain weight almost over night. My metabolism simply shuts down leaving me feeling tired, groggy, and bloated. Even through I may cheat at times I continue to strive toward perfection. If I eat cooked foods I make sure to add something fresh. As fresh fruit and vegetables are filled with digestive enzymes, I always try to add a fresh piece of fruit or salad items, which might include onions, tomatoes, or other vegetables.

During my trip to Jeanerette I experienced this imbalance for the first time. I was drinking a large amount of diet drinks artificially sweetened with aspartame along with some other weight control ingredients. This caused a physical as well as a psychological imbalance in my system. To combat this imbalance, I increased my soy intake. Rather than taking a soy pill in an effort to obtain the complete nutrients, I ate soy nuts daily. Also including certain natural soy protein bars, as well as made my soy and rice protein shake along with extra vitamin C, E, B-complex, and one chewable or liquid multiple vitamin supplement. As I have found some liquids, powders, or chewable vitamins made from a whole food may be more a more absorbable form. I learned this fact first hand after giving my mother certain pills, I noted they went in and came out in the same whole form. And after a few weeks and lots of prayer, I began to regain a healthy state of being.

&&&&&&&

Nutritional Notes:
Basically fresh fruit should be eaten alone, especially melons to avoid the meal turning in into acid. I further try to eat only multi-whole grains such as cereals that include brown rice, buckwheat, rye, sesame, and quinoa. I also eat lots of soybeans such as tofu and meat substitute products such as veggie-burgers. Soy is great for the body and naturally helps overall health of an imbalance in the body's system or rather imbalanced hormones. As I strive to reach my goals, I sometimes become complacent and start to pick the weight up again. So in an effort to continue my quest, I further figured my ideal weight based on my height. It is called body mass index or BMI, it's calculated by weight in kilograms divided by height in meters squared, [BMI = (weight in pounds x 700) divided by (height in inches$^2$). A BMI of 25 to 30 is considered overweight, and over 30 may be considered obese. Realizing that I had lost forty pounds just a couple of years before, I knew once I took off the weight this time I could not let this continue to happen time and time again. The main consideration or guidelines I wanted to avoid was a crash diet. I preferred to change my eating habits rather than fad diets, and as I age I had to be cautious as well as I needed help. I needed to stick with my sound diet as well as fast and pray for help. I continued my teas such as cleansing teas with dandelion, red clover, milk thistle, and added ginkgo biloba and lemongrass tea to help metabolize fat.

I further temporarily added supplements to help metabolize fat with, L-Carnitine, vitamin E, a supplement with high B-complex nutrients such as choline, which are all good for the brain as well. Also I added extra biotin to help breakdown proteins along with folic acid, and ester C. Coenzyme 10, maitake or shitake mushrooms, proteolytic enzymes with bromelain or garlic and enzymes all support the immune system response which includes fibroid tumor growth and inflammation. Proteolytic enzymes aid in the body's digestion to help prevent as well as break down formation of cell abnormally and growths. Flax seed oil also assist with proper cell formation as well. Some other supplements include zinc lozenges, a little chromium picolinate that also help maintain healthy blood sugar level, while herbs like garcinia cambogia tea has worked wonders for suppressing my appetite keeping the carbohydrates from metabolizing into fat. Fenugreek has a sweet syrup consistency and can be great as a tea or seasoning. It helps mucous build up, asthma, sinus and lung problems, fever, eyes, intestines, and simulates a bulk laxative. Furthermore, I sometimes add aloe vera and apple juice or a tablespoon of apple cider vinegar to about eight ounces of water at bedtime two or three times during the week.

*As I advocate a whole and natural foods diet, if I want to snack I love NOW brand cajun or barbecue seasoned soybeans as well as kashi whole grain cereal with rice and/or soymilk combination.* Kashi is filled with fiber and nutrients and is a wonderful nutritionally sound snack. But as I am trying to loose weight, I try to limit my food intake. Also, gymestra sylvestra helps destroy excess sugar while lowering cholesterol.

Amino acids such as L-Carnitine or sometimes L-Tyrosine help reduce my body fat. I have also sometimes taken L-Arginine, which can retard tumor growth, along with L-Ornithine and L-Lysine for muscle tone. As I do not practice taking separate amino's because too much of one amino without the others can cause problems. For example, too much L-Arginine and L-Orthinine without L-Lysine can cause an imbalance in your system creating a state of confusion. Amino acids are the building block of proteins and can be basically derived from whey, a complete protein that contains all the amino acids, or a vegetarian complete protein. Also you can combine beans with rice and corn, to obtain all essential amino's which constitutes a complete protein. Also you can combine nuts as well. Nuts are also a good source for not only vitamins but protein as well.

Other protein sources include meat such as turkey and salmon, milk, yogurt, or cholesterol free tofu to name a few. Your protein should equal around half your body weight in grams, such as a person who weighs about 140 pounds should intake about 50 to 70 grams of daily protein for proper body functions. Also a vegetable protein drink with spirulina, chlorella, kelp, alfalfa, barley, rice bran, royal jelly, FOS such as acidophilus provide healthy intestinal bacteria, and other great ingredients are a better choice for providing your amino's than taking them separately, spirulina, a green algae also assist in weight management. I try not to take various separate amino acids as they can cause complications such as too much phenylalanine, which has been linked to tumor growth. Also, herbs such as ephedra or ma hung have been known to have adverse affects such as causing heart problems.

⌘ ⌘ ⌘ ⌘ ⌘ ⌘ ⌘ ⌘ ⌘ ⌘

## *Early 2001*

As I continue to fight the fight for good health, I was further living with a deviated septum that was inhibiting my breathing from my first car accident at age nineteen as I hit my chin on the steering wheel. I then developed what was termed TMJ (tempormandibular joint) problems causing an inflamed jaw joint. My jaw would often pop as I would open and close my mouth, and a lump that surfaced on my neck were all injuries that stemmed from the car accident trauma. Although the lump on my neck was benign the ENT doctor advised if I opted to correct the deviated septum through surgery, I could in fact have the knot on my neck removed at the same time. I knew I was having difficulty breathing at night and sometimes during the day and probably needed it. But I would opt to wait until I had more time to heal, as my life did not allow time for yet another surgery.

Nutritional Notes:

When I make time for the spa I exercise by using the bikes and some of the various machines for my problem area. Also as I exercise by tightening my muscles, inhaling, and slowly releasing the tightened muscles as I exhale. *I knew appropriate oxygen flow helps the body heal as I practiced deep breathing exercises as often as possible.* Deep breathing exercise can be done in the car by while driving or even lying in bed. In the car I carefully tighten my abdomen, arms, or backside while inhaling through my nose for as long as I can, and then releasing or blowing the breathe out for almost twice as long. While in bed I lye flat with my toes pointing toward the top of my body, which pulls the back leg muscles as do leg lifts. Then I further tighten my thighs, abdomen, and body while inhaling through the nose and releasing through the mouth. Again the breathes are long but my exhales are longer, as this is a good early morning wake up before getting ready for work. As I like to do at least ten repetitions, but the number of repetitions depends on how early I wake up for work. Another daily morning exercise I try to do is while lying flat on my back with my legs bent and feet flat, my elbows are used to support my upper body while my hands rest in my lower back. I then lift my pelvic up while tilting my head back similar to standing on your head for as long as possible for several repetitions. Also when I cannot get to the gym I continue exercising by doing leg lifts, stretches, jumping jacks, and taking the stairs at least seven to eleven flights a day as I continue to believe my body will be totally healed with exercise and proper diet.

In an effort to maintain proper diet I sometimes try to do a juice fast for at least of days. It not only gives your digestive system a rest, but also helps to cleanse your system. Carrot, cranberry and/or blueberry, grapefruit, orange, beets, with apple juice and/or cantaloupe to help burn fat and cleanse my system along with my vitamins and I sometimes include a high protein drink. Another diet I had good results with is my soup-cleansing program, which heals and cleanses the system. I also included some meal suggestions, which can provide needed nutrition while the soup is cleansing the body. Cruciferous vegetables such as cauliflower, kale, broccoli, and brussel sprouts cleanses the colon and helps prevent tumor and cancer growths, celery and parsley cleanses also and can provide the needed chlorophyll to help detoxify the body. Apple juice will help remove the heavy metal toxins, and if you just eat soup only I attempt a three-day limit. As this soup cleanses your body of various toxic body conditions, it also removes needed vitamins and minerals. I try to restore these nutrients by including some nutrient rich meal suggestions along with an all natural whole food vitamin and mineral supplement. Although meat is considered acidic, meat including beef supplies the body with some needed nutrients such as B12. Therefore, if I decide not to eat meat such as steak, I try to include extra B12 as well as B complex.

SOUP RECIPE: LOTS OF GARLIC, ONIONS, CARROTS, CAULIFLOWER, CELERY, KALE, BEETS, PARSLEY, TURNIP (SMALL), WATER IN A LARGE POT (OPTIONAL 1 TO 2 CUPS ORGANIC APPLE JUICE) AND LOTS OF HERBAL SEASONINGS. SOUP CAN BE EATEN AS OFTEN AS YOU LIKE. PLEASE NOTE THIS SOUP IS KNOWN TO HEAL THE BODY AND PREVENT THE ONSET OF ILLNESS, BUT TAKE A GOOD HEALTH FOOD STORE MULTIVITAMIN/MINERAL (PREFERABLY FROM A WHOLE FOOD SOURCE).

## 7-Day Soup Cleansing with Meal Suggestions

| DAY ONE: FRUIT | *BREAKFAST* | *LUNCH* | *DINNER* |
|---|---|---|---|
| Meal Suggestions: | CANTALOUPE | WATERMELON | WATERMELON |
| | 3 8OZ GLASSES | 3 8OZ GLASSES | WATERMELON |
| | OF WATER | OF WATER | SOUP |
| | | SOUP | 2 8OZ GLASSES OF WATER |
| DAY TWO: Vegetables | *BREAKFAST* | *LUNCH* | *DINNER* |
| Meal Suggestions: | TOMATOES | GREENS | GREENS |
| | 3 8OZ GLASSES | SWEET POTATO | MUSHROOMS |
| | OF WATER | SOUP | SOUP |
| | | 3 GLASSES WATER | 2 GLASSES WATER |
| DAY THREE: Fruit & Vegetables | *BREAKFAST* | *LUNCH* | *DINNER* |
| Meal Suggestions: | WATERMELON | FRUIT | FRUIT |
| | 3 GLASSES WATER | GREENS | VEGETABLES |
| | | SOUP | SOUP |
| | | 3 GLASSES WATER | 2 GLASSES WATER |
| DAY FOUR: | *BREAKFAST* | *LUNCH* | *DINNER* |
| Meal Suggestions: | 3 BANANAS | 2 BANANAS | 3 BANANAS |
| | Low Carb High Protein | Low Carb High Protein | Low Carb High Protein Drink |
| | 3 GLASSES WATER | SOUP | SOUP |
| | | 3 GLASSES WATER | 2 GLASSES OF WATER |
| DAY FIVE: Vegetables & Meat | *BREAKFAST* | *LUNCH* | *DINNER* |
| Meal Suggestions: | 5 OZ STEAK OR | 5 OZ STEAK OR | 5 OZ STEAK OR |
| | MEAT EQUIVALENT | MEAT EQUIVALENT | MEAT EQUIVALENT |
| | 2 TOMATOES | 2 TOMATOES | 2 TOMATOES |
| | 3 GLASSES WATER | 3 GLASSES WATER | 2 GLASSES WATER |
| | | SOUP | SOUP |
| DAY SIX: Meat & Vegetables | *BREAKFAST* | *LUNCH* | *DINNER* |
| Meal Suggestions: | TOMATOES | 5 OZ STEAK OR | 5 OZ STEAK OR |
| | 3 GLASSES WATER | MEAT EQUIVALENT | MEAT EQUIVALENT |
| | | GREENS | KALE |
| | | BROCCOLI | GREENS |
| | | SOUP | SOUP |
| | | 3 GLASSES WATER | 2 GLASSES WATER |
| DAY SEVEN: Fruit & Vegetables | *BREAKFAST* | *LUNCH* | *DINNER* |
| Meal Suggestions: | FRUIT | GREENS//SOUP | BROWN RICE/SOUP |
| | BROWN RICE/SOUP | BROCCOLI | GREENS |

| 3 GLASSES WATER | 1 PIECE ORGANIC FRUIT | TOMATOES |
| | | 1 PIECE ORGANIC FRUIT |
| | 3 GLASSES WATER | 2 GLASSES WATER |

*Also, one might think that since there are a large amount acidic foods in the meal suggestion, but most fresh fruits and vegetables are not considered acid forming foods. But if you do want to find out if your body is to acidic or alkaline which both cause illness purchase pH paper in the pharmacy and apply saliva or urine. Too much acid can cause an imbalance and contribute to cravings leading to weight gain. Acidic foods include all foods with added sugar such as junk foods and sodas, meats, coffee, tea, cocoa, pepper, eggs, shellfish, alcohol, catsup, sauerkraut, aspirin, tobacco, most drugs, and noodles just to mention a few. To maintain body balance one should add alkaline foods such as honey, avocados, corn, most fresh fruits and vegetables, maple syrup, molasses, raisins, and soy products. Although this diet contains food such as kale, turnips, and broccoli, which contain some alkalizing mineral content most fresh fruits and vegetables are not considered acid forming foods. I did add an extra food source for additional calcium and magnesium. Hence, granulated kelp can be used as seasoning and is high in mineral content and can aid creating an alkaline body. Taking good absorbable magnesium, calcium supplement such as kelp can assist any needed mineral content. Also make sure your water is purified pH balanced or distilled which is one of the purest forms of absorbable water.*

❊ ❊ ❊ ❊ ❊ ❊ ❊ ❊ ❊ ❊ ❊ ❊ ❊ ❊

About one year later after all my proper diet concerns, I returned to the ENT doctor for my septum or rather sinus surgery as well as removal of the small knot on my neck. But due to all the changes in my diet the knot on my neck had gotten tremendously smaller. The doctor advised it was so small it was not worth removing and only performed the septum surgery. Also I try to continue to take care of myself, and have come to the realization that otherwise, I would be unable to care for my mother. Although Helen as well as myself may continue to have our bouts of ailment setbacks, I continue to move toward my natural nutritional concepts. I proceed with more diligence since natural does not always mean a nutritionally sound product. We are both continuing to heal our wounds from our mostly fresh fruit and vegetable regiment as well as our other dietary changes and supplements. I continue to give her natural anti-inflammatory supplements such as querctin and/or bromelin (found in pineapple) for her throat and digestive tract, which sometimes narrows causing an inability to swallow food, as she use to merely chew the food removing most of the juice substance and then spit it out.  The swollen and pus pockets in her legs are only a shadow in our memories as it has been completely cured.  The diverticulitus is virtually healed as the episodes of bleeding from the mouth as well as the rectum have almost ceased.  Helen's rheumatoid arthritis is gradually healing, as she does not suffer with extreme pain when the weather changes to rainy or cold.

But I still found myself running up and down the steps trying to get her comfortable to no avail.  I would previously go back and forth, turning her, as well as whole body rubdowns with lotion I had bought as well as my homemade ones.  I can never be completely positive, but this time I am sure it played an important part in relieving her painful stroke symptoms.  After the stroke I found myself trying to figure out what was hurting her, as her speech remains very slurred.  I eventually learned that pain occurs with a stroke from regaining feeling in the affected limbs.  Now after about eight months she has began to sleep through the night, although she continues to have bouts of digestive ailments, which I attempted to try to keep under control.  First, I would call her neurologists as I thought it might be related to the medications, but he advised to call her general practitioner.  After much frustration and getting little help from her neurologist and her general doctors, as I suppose they were doing the best they could, I just continued to read.  I tried to give her more bulk such as insoluble fiber and a nutritional vegetarian protein drink supplement as everything she would eat was pureed, I felt it might help balance her system and it did.

Although I still might sometimes have go back and forth checking on her as she moans in pain, because she needs changing or just can't sleep I still continued to thank God because I knew she was doing better.  As she once came back from mass confusion and hallucinations, I have regained the faith once again believing she will be healed from the stroke and memory loss once more.

I feel God had worked before and he can do it again in this situation.  As he has worked miracles over and over again in my life, I would have been motherless a long time ago.  I thank the Lord and Savior Jesus Christ for sparing both our lives.  As I think back on how I would whine about how Helen continued to forget as she would even sometimes forget we moved into a new house. As she always wanted to leave and return home, or ask the same question right after I would answer. But now after her stroke and we were unable to have any meaning communication, I sometimes wish she could ask me a question over and over again. The stroke has further rendered her unable to feed herself or tell you when she has to use the bathroom. While I try to stay in silent prayer for her condition to get better, I do thank God she is still here for me to feed, as I began to see my views on compassion continue to reach higher heights.

As my mother continued to have the TIA's I found myself sometimes pacing, rather than sitting in the emergency room most of the night. I still continued my research in hopes she would get better once again. I further would make suggestions to her doctors as I inquired about cholesterol lowering drugs, although her cholesterol was 165 I thought we could have looked into obtaining an even lower reading such as 120 with medication. I further mentioned to the doctor for possible consideration of hyperbaric (oxygen treatment) as he merely advised it was not being used for stroke treatment. I had read in one of my books that it was a consideration to help with brain healing after stroke infractions. The neurologist exclaimed her condition was merely a part aging, because as we age the arteries harden.

As I had recently learned the TIA's or mini strokes are considered a precursor to a massive stroke, I would request the doctor to order an oxygen machine for the house just in case I ever needed it. Little did I know that I would need it sooner than I thought as the saga that was about to unfold would cause my mother to need it regularly.

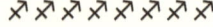

*Late 2001/Early 2002*

As I try to monitor her condition regularly, I made a decision to feed her pureed organic baby foods which included a regiment of one jar of prunes in the morning mixed with some powdered vitamins and brown rice syrup.  I still gave cooked her egg substitute with culinary seasonings, 1 part rice or soy milk, fig and raspberry rice bars, rice bran, and ½ cup tea.  Other baby foods I sometimes included were organic beans and brown rice, corn, and for lunch with other organic fruits, and sometimes organic pureed turkey at night.  Then as her frequent hospital visits slowed, I was able to start back cooking split peas, whole grain quinoa, steamed vegetables and used the leftovers from her juicer as fiber, and pureed corn for her complete protein. I further included pureed macadamia and cashew nut butter with added juice or water, organic royal jelly in honey, a tablespoon of olive oil, and brown rice bran for added fiber, nutrition, and extra calories. These foods provided a smoother consistency for her pureed diet. I further concluded and continue to note considerations in her diet plans.

*Mid 2002*

During all my new found dietary information breakthroughs, Helen further continued to take her plavix for the sticking blood platelets. At night I sometimes give her additional magnesium asporate or orotate totaling at least 1000 milligrams daily and a little calcium. Although I sometimes wish I had continued her on her chondroitin combination, bromelin, enzymes, B-6, and zinc for her bone and arthritis nutritional supplement.  This was not only an anti-inflammatory, but help build and sustain her muscles including the esophagus as well as the heart. But when she first had the massive stroke I gave her a calcium chloride blend, as it is good for the heart, which I recently started again.  Also during her restless nights I included a little melatonin, skullcap and valerian combination along with melatonin as they are considered nervine herbs and contribute to restful sleep.

Then I thought she might be leaving us after a couple of close calls.
The first afternoon incident was during lunch, and Helen simply started
to gag while I was feeding her some salmon.  Then she just stopped
breathing and while I frantically called for my son to call 911, I thought
she might have been choking.  Hence, as I yelled for help to Joseph,
"Help, Help, tell them to come she's dying. Please come, Please she's
dying. Joseph help me," as I continued to perform the Heimlich
maneuver.  Finally after what seemed to be an hour but realistically
probably about five minutes, Helen was breathing again. The ambulance
took her to a new hospital in the area, but they released her only for her
to return a few days later with the exact same scenario.  The next
occurrence the home health aide performed CPR, while she was bleeding
from her rectum profusely.  This time I took her to a hospital where her
regular physician is resident, and as she laid in the emergency room
waiting it looked like I was about to loose her.  I pleaded with them to
quickly give her some blood.  Eventually after a few pints of blood and
her doctor's assistance, the bleeding stopped within a couple of days as
she had been taking the plavix pretty regularly.  Her survival through this
ordeal was certainly another miracle.

Then after Helen's continued TIA's, restless nights, continued loose
bowels,  and the bleeding incident I took her off plavix,  the blood
thinner.  I started to give her the aspirin only.  I further decided to take
her off the arthritic medication and will always regret putting her back on
this medication in the first place as it had been linked to heart attack and
stroke.

Not long after she had a third attack but without the bleeding, after
describing how stiff her body and neck was the visiting nurse as well as
the ambulance driver advised it was probably caesuras.  As they
sometimes occur after a massive stroke and the doctor could prescribe a
mild medication to help control the attacks.  In the meantime while I was
trying to obtain a caesurae medication from her doctor, she had yet
another attack.

This time they diagnosed it as another TIA and I would later learn
after requesting her hospital records that the doctor further added some
signs of malnutrition and dehydration.  Her doctor started to recommend

a feeding tube. I thought how could she be malnutrition and dehydrated as I sat her meals out and water out for the daytime caregiver who stays with my mother. I started to seriously doubt myself and change her regiment once again, and discontinuing certain things one of which I feel was vital to her cell regeneration including the IP-6 hexanicotinate, quinoa, split peas, flax seed, chondroitin, phosphatidylserine, and GABA for the brain, as I started give her more baby food. Finally, I found it could be a reality as the daily caretakers changed frequently, and I started to find some of hidden jars of baby food in places I did not put it. The doctor felt her water intake could be increased as well, thereby possibly helping to circumvent these attacks. But I knew this should not be the case as I asked the caretakers on a daily basis to give all of her water, as well as asking them to let me know the amount of water she actually drank.

Although I was reluctant, I finally decided to allow this procedure, as it appeared to be the most logical solution to the problem. But my eldest brother found it unacceptable, as he knew just I that Helen always was adamantly against any type of surgery, which included any and all types of procedures. In the past my mother walked away from hospitals and doctors she trusted dearly, refusing everything from a simple scope of her stomach and digestive system to diverticulitis surgery. As I had signed for more procedures than my mother had in her whole lifetime, my brother's action was no doubt a gentle reminder of my mother's wishes as I began to feel much guilt for what I had already allowed. Furthermore after considering all of my mother's previous stomach problems including an obstruction, ulcers from arthritis medications, as well as bleeding, she might not have tolerated this type of surgery. Later on I would even further appreciate my brother's decision, as this hospital almost took her life from infection.

Out of all Helen's past problems including the stroke, she was still alert attempting to communicate and still trying sing. For the most part she generally did pretty good after her massive stroke, and considering all she had been through and her age. She loved to sing her old gospel songs, but would never be the same after this hospital stay. This hospital visit turned into a month long nightmare as they continued to have much difficulty locating and keeping the IV in her vein. The IV leaked into her arm several times overnight, as I would have to check on her at least three times a day. As I would have to go by the hospital every morning on my way to work and feed Helen, morning visits was when I would find her arms larger than her thighs, as well as blisters on her arms and hands from the IV fluids leaking. The fluid literally invaded her whole body, as I pleaded with the nurses to discontinue the IV. As I complained to the hospital administration mainly that staff was neglecting to check the IV throughout the night, but this would only backfire.

One night I requested them to weigh Helen and her weight was at least twenty to thirty pounds over her normal weight. I pleaded with the nurse to stop the IV that night before I left. I even called back throughout that night, but the head nurse refused to turn off the IV stating the doctor would have to approve it and she refused to call the doctor. Finally, when I walked in the next morning I found my mother gasping for breath. She almost went into a deadly cardiac arrest, I was terrified, but one LVN advised she had cut off the IV, notified the respiratory therapy for breathing treatments, and called the doctor to order some lasix to help remove the IV fluid overload. Again in the midst of disaster, one small light beamed down and saved us once again. Although Helen would never be the same after this hospital stay, it was a light of joy to know God's angel still walk among the earth watching and saving lives just when needed as he sent this LVN to save her that day.

But I felt so bad about this hospital visit, as what started as a minor visit for a TIA turned into a thirty-day stay. As she even developed an infection while she was there and they were so irresponsible, and the IV continued to leak into her body overnight. The hospital administration eventually decided to call AP Services on me for not doing the feeding tube in a continued effort to retaliate against my complaints, and in an attempt to cover their mistakes against any lawsuits. As the APS representative with this most unfounded illegitimate claim greeted me, she advised I could report the hospital as well to the state board for the bad care my mother received. But I knew that this hospital could not be

entrusted with surgical procedures as Helen had already developed
continued infection from the IV leaking.

The saga continued to play out as Helen returned again to yet
another hospital within a couple of weeks.  The attending emergency
room physician immediately put her on lasix to remove excess fluid as
the previous visit was still haunting us.  Finally, a cardiologist diagnosed
her with a mild heart attack and prescribed a nitroglycerine patch that I
still continue to sometimes use for her enlarged heart condition.  Little
did I know at the time that the excessive IV fluids leaking into her organs
from the previous hospital neglect were the causation factor for this
initial attack and ongoing continued problems and would ultimately
plummet into even more serious catastrophes, as she had to remain on
the breathing treatments until her untimely death.

During all the tragic hospital stays and allegations, I decided to
prepare all Helen's meals as well as put her vitamins in the food.
Measuring out her daily amount of water and leaving everything on the
counter top before I left for work.  I further asked the sitters to leave any
food or water even if it was a spoonful in the refrigerator, as we needed
to count her calories

Then she started to exhibit a little blood in her stool and I took back
once more to the nearest hospital that had previously put her on the nitro
and lasix, and further requested a gastrologist to examine her. The
gastrologist was able to stop the rectal bleeding and as Helen had started
to eat rather slowly she suggested a feeding tube but I refused. They put
her into the intensive care unit and the head nurse shut the curtain on me,
and advised me to wait outside as she tried time after time to insert an IV
as I clenched in dismay as my mother moaned and groaned from the
needle sticking her.  Finally I walked in the room as I had enough, and
she called in a technician to complete the procedure. She was extremely
overbearing as she moved and readjusted or moved every pillow I put in
place for my mother. As I tried to make her feel better after all of the
needle sticks to my mother by making conversation and apologizing to
her for walking back in the room, she made no remarks and just ignored
me

The next day the nurse called me at work and stated the staff doctor requested approval to do a procedure because he felt she was still bleeding from somewhere.  By the time I arrived at the hospital my mother was so distraught and unresponsive, as the staff doctor must have given her some type of anesthesia during the procedure.  I tried to find out what happened but the doctor became especially defensive. As my mother's physical mental condition appeared severely comprised, I knew this doctor must have given her some type of unwarranted medication that was not necessary for a person in her condition.  I inquired about the procedure with the nurse by advising how I thought the gastrologist previously examined her for bleeding. I further stated what was he going to do if he found any bleeding. But she could not respond, as he did not even locate any bleeding.  I thought what was his purpose for calling me at work requesting permission for performing this procedure, and all I could think about was how Helen always thought some of her doctors were merely experimenting on her. This staff doctor further threatened to call APS in retaliation of my complaints, and to cover his self for performing this unwarranted procedure since my mother was virtually unresponsive.  As I went home with Hospice I felt he knew exactly what he did incorrectly, and feared the worst.

As she continued exhibited minimal swallowing difficulty but did continue to have hospital visits from congestive heart failure, the new caregiver we hired was feeding her and she appeared to be doing well during the day for the most part.  So I remained true to her wishes of not wanting to have any surgery.  And this no doubt requires lots of continued prayer, research and reading, lots of unwavering dedication, and continued work.  But I always thank God for the opportunity to be able to serve and assist her.

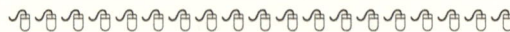

<u>*Late 2003*</u>:

As my son Joseph has gotten older and sometimes assists me with my mother, hugging her continually telling her that he loves her. And when I am unable to get her to cooperate, Joseph sometimes helps just by talking and laughing.  Although we do not know if she understands, she does still have feelings and no doubt understands that love is around her as she laughs with Joseph.  Joseph is such a loving child as he always says, "I love you", and if I do not return the phrase quick enough he says, " Ma, you don't know what might happen.  That's why we should always say I love you to each other".  Joseph will always be one of my gentle reminders that love and family is the most important gift in the world.

I also constantly received continued praise from everyone my family, friends, to even co-workers on how I really have done a wonderful job in taking care of my ailing mother, as my mother had not been in good health for over the last fifteen years.  She was in and out of the emergency room and hospital mostly for her diverticulitis and poor circulation.  But lately I started to impress upon myself to do better, and worried about Helen constantly.  I felt God impressing upon my spirit to do a fast, but during this time and over the past year I had not been eating or exercising properly and it became extremely difficult to continue a fast.  As I unconsciously raced against the clock to make her better, between all the sometimes very tolling hospital stays.  Then after her last stay in the hospital she would develop bad bedsores, and this last doctor appeared to do very little to help her as well as ignore my suggestions as I would constantly remind him of her congestive heart failure and maybe he should call in a specialist.  Hence, because of this I was hesitant on her staying in the hospital under his care and asked for her release. When she returned from the hospital, her daily caregiver decided to work weekends only.  In my haste I decided to let one of the ladies return who had previously cared for my mother on the weekends only to come back on the weekdays, her returning caregiver advised me she was eating and doing fine during the day.  Then about week and half later, the weekend caregiver advised it appeared something was wrong with my mother's left side around her rib cage appeared swollen. I asked everyday and even called throughout the day inquiring on what occurred and on how Helen was doing, her daily caregiver advised she was eating all her food and again doing fine.  Then I noticed it appeared she was losing weight, my initial thought was possibly that it was just maybe because she was not getting enough water during the day, but I was giving her water at night.  The caregiver stated she was eating all her food, but in the past the other caregiver would always have something leftover that I had to finish.  But now I realize I may have been to trusting and did not respond quick enough.

We had so much going on at work with a systems upgrade project which required a lot of time, concentration, dealing with varying personalities, and perceptions of dedication while installing piecemeal incremental inept system enhancements.  I transferred to this department right after Helen's stroke in year 2000 and eventually moved to this particular section after about a year.  I do not think anyone really understood how sick my mother really was during this time, and one slip up could in fact cost the ultimate price.  Working through lunch breaks and late evenings while my motives were being questioned, as I had to mainly leave on time to get home and care for my mother.  This added additional stress to my already stressed situation.  I just could not even think straight as I was being pulled in too many unwarranted directions and I asked my manager to be transferred to no avail.  I added a screen saver on my computer, " Jesus Loves You" as a reminder to keep the faith and strength.  I further tried reading the bible during breaks.

Meanwhile my son had his school functions or interests, and I will never live down the fact that I missed his first starring role in his theatrical play after which he stood alone outside waiting for me to pick him up.  Tears just stream down my face as all I can say to him is I am sorry, and try to explain that it is a huge and difficult responsibility trying to take care of a household alone.  As a single parent I try to instill in him to be the best he can be no matter what the circumstances may entail that surround you.  No matter what situation you may be born in you must strife for success not only to set an example but also be in a position to help others, who may find themselves in a most unfortunate situation.  All these events would now only be mere precursors to what was about to unfold.

I was so distraught with the hospital as I felt they were the cause of Helens' congestive heart problems, and every time she went in she would get unbelievable bedsores.  It would take me months to get hem back under control.  I guess I had gotten tired of those places just as my mother. But I knew we needed to get the most recent bedsore under control very quickly, from the moment Helen returned from her last hospital stay, I would request the nurse practitioner who did home visits for the doctor to come by but to no avail as there was always a conflict in her schedule. I was also calling the visiting nurses daily who cared for her bedsore to come by daily, and finally after requesting an emergency visit, a nurse came out over on the weekend and advised I should take her back to the hospital. Finally her regular nurse came back out immediately afterwards, the following Monday, and said she appeared alert and doing well and ordered some medication for her sore.

But for some reason on that Tuesday night she became less responsive I decided to take her into the hospital on Wednesday. But as the caregiver came in and I was already running late for work that morning I decided to wait until latter that day. But I waited one day too late, as I rushed out of the house to work. Not even a few minutes after I arrived at work the sitter called me and said Helen stop breathing as she just walked out of the room for a moment. But she had called the paramedics and they had her back breathing. I was devastated as I asked to speak to the paramedics, they advised she was not breathing when they arrived, and they were still unable to revive her. A few days later the nurse called for me to pick up the medication for her as well as the doctor's home visiting service finally called me back with an appointment, and to their surprise I would advise both she had died.

I will never know exactly what happened that morning, but it appears my worst nightmare had become reality. The ultimate reason why I took Helen out of the nursing home was fear of her not being taken care of. As I looked back and recalled not long after Helen's massive stroke I started to feel a spiritual time in my heart of seven years that I could not completely understand at the time. Now it would become a reality. My first thought was ultimately a time frame of grace added to Helen's life after all her stroke. As I continued to try to rely on my own understanding rather than my spiritual understanding, as I began to hear things in my heart. Thoughts such as God can allow Helen to live to be ninety or even beyond, which may have been true. These thoughts would overshadow the reality that she lived seven years from the time I started this healing quest despite what the doctors thought and did.

She had been thriving for years only by the miraculous, especially after the hospital stay where the IV fluids leaked all over her body. Her body was so large and her arms were swollen from the IV to about the size of her thighs and I further feel these fluids invaded the lungs, as they had to administer lasix. She further required oxygen along with breathing treatments, which we had to continue until her untimely passing. Other organs in her body were compromised as she was prescribed nitroglycerine as well. Further the hospital visit that gave her anesthesia to scope her for bleeding, without my written consent, compromised her health even more. It was not any surprise that I dreaded the days I had to take her back to the hospital, and while trying to continue to honor her wishes not wanting surgery. I basically developed a general distrust of most of the medical community, and will always feel this hospital visit was the initial cause of my mother's early demise. All of the subsequent visits after this one were always related to her heart and breathing problems. As it appeared it was merely through God's grace that she would always return home from her many hospital stays. I knew living through all this as most do not at her age, and further recall that even down through the years how some of her doctors sent her home over the pass seven years anticipating her survival rate to be less than six months. But she lived seven and years beyond since her initial diagnosis with life threatening conditions.

Also a few weeks before Helen passed a small clock in my restroom, that I received as a token award from one of my jobs for perfect attendance, started to beep. But it started to go off just out of the blue about 5am every morning. I even tried to shut off the clock by putting the switch in the off alarm position, but it still continued to go off. I could only imagine that it might have been God's way of telling me that either something was wrong, or it was time to give my mother a rest from this life as she moved toward her next life with him in heaven.

While this may be a new day with new and great breakthroughs and inventions of mankind, it is still also a day with even more grave concern.  Concern for the integrity of the medical communities proper training, procedural guidelines, and appropriate communication.

While I was so busy listening to what I should and could do, I sometimes feel I literally missed on the final hours of my mother's care. Then, I finally received a revelation that in life certain events may sometimes happen, which includes the good and well intention people. These events more often than not have nothing to do with your level of education or your level of intelligence.  As I thought the more educated professionals such as doctors, lawyers, nurses, judges, etc., sometimes never miss the key objective and make mistakes.  But the fact remains we are all only human and maybe I did not follow the path that the medical community thought I should, and maybe the medical community such as doctors, nurses, administrators as well as her caregivers did not follow the appropriate procedure.  The only difference is negligence and willful intent, and although I do feel the medical community might have encompassed some willful negligence which contributed to her early demise, I further feel my dedication to care for my to care for my mother and honoring her wishes was all I could do.  I depended on myself to provide her nutrition, but I also depended on others to provide appropriate care as well.  Now I know I did all the Lord above would let me do, nothing more and nothing less and it was the very best I could considering all the circumstances.  Maybe if the hospital and others I trusted would had worked with me, instead of against me, my mother would still be here.  Communication is a delicate thing and sometimes when procedures are not followed, patients are put on the back burner. All logical reasoning and communication is blocked by the negligence, which causes you to loose faith in just about everyone in the system. And that is what happened in my situation, as I was caring for my mother often times I was told what I should do most abruptly, and if I did not comply I was viewed as the enemy.  As hospitals poked and peddled needles and scopes in my mother, and I further I entrusted others to care for her during the day it was no doubt out of my control.

I feel that God's holy spirit reveals to us what to pray for and just maybe this time was her time.  Although I know my mother was ready a long time ago, I just have to move past what the final hours or circumstances may entail even though I may wish it had turned out very differently.

    I further recall not long after my father passed, Helen told us of a dream in which she was extraordinarily awaken with a phone call about four o'clock in the morning. The dream was in a beautiful garden with lovely flowers, trees, a waterfall, and bridge. As my mother stood on one side of the bridge, on the other side was my father reaching out his hand motioning and persuading her to come across. At that moment she started across the phone would ring and it was my brother Fred who to this day does not know why he telephoned her at such an early hour. But not long after that incident my mother started to let us know she was preparing to go, as she would mention it quite frequently over the last twenty years. As we tried to change the subject and lighten the mood, she persisted envisioning a burial of light blue and chiffon.

    Caring for my mother has no doubt taught me that in life there are still God's angels walking with us and we must learn to discern their voices. Sometimes I feel as though if I had just stayed with what appeared to work from the onset, but I continued to research further and further trying to completely cure her, while continuing to doubt myself. Not fully realizing what may have been occurring right before my eyes. When she was doing well and I had good people caring for her that was a miracle in itself.

    Although I was able to acquire an enormous amount of knowledge, this total experience in my life has resulted in my renewed sense that I do not want to miss hearing the voice of God. Human beings make mistakes and will continue to repeat the same mistakes unless we hear and obey the powerful spiritual voice inside us. We do not have the strength on our own to overcome adversities, but through the powerful son and Savoir Jesus, whom we can do all things. I do not believe this was a coincidence and by far the most important legacy my mother would want to leave with me.

    As it became clear to me whatever you desire in life you must first give in order to receive.

    *If you want Gods attention, you must first give him attention by listening to his still soft voice, his angels still walk among us and we*

*must learn to discern their voices when we sometimes cannot discern for*
*ourselves. Maybe we can save a life if we just take time to listen and*
*obey. As I felt God had been imparting upon my spirit to fast and pray,*
*but it just seemed as though I was too stressed to obey.*

In consideration of everything that occurred over the pass seven
years, and after beating up on myself for the past few days after Helen's
death I decided to do something out of the ordinary but most significant
to me. Maybe it would assist in my attempt to become a better person, as
I needed to leave some of the negative past and thoughts behind. Finally
after much debate I reminded myself of a biblical story of Saul, who
changed his name to Paul after becoming renewed and an eventual Saint,
as I was trying to renew a meaning life I decided to change my first
name.

Although I feel I could never be compared to Paul by any means,
I do feel that just maybe I can continue to do and live like God has
intended, as I wanted to learn how to hear and discern his spiritual voice.
Although changing a name is superficial and does not change a mind,
heart, or soul of the person, I am hoping and praying I will regain my life
one day because at this point I have loss my will to continue as normal.
Nothing is normal any more and no longer is it business as usual, but
rather feelings of sorrow consume me once more. As I often feel I
should have reacted differently to this ongoing saga, as almost all who
was involved in her care during her final months caused me to doubt
everything I was doing for my mother.

I now ask the Lord to help me discern his will and desires for my
life, as I do not want to miss the will of God, because missing it could
mean the difference between being in the wrong place with the wrong
people, peace or confusion, and ultimately the difference between life or
death.

But I did miss him once more as my brother Charles would pass
barely two years after my mother. We all knew he probably took my
mother's death the most difficult, as I know we were all equally as hurt.
I pleaded with his wife to let him live as I believed he would get better,
she refused and sided with the hospital after barely a week in ICU. I was
devastated once more. I cringed with despair as I recently had a vision of

my brother healed and speaking of his miracle at Lakewood Church with his entire family present, as Joel's mother asked him to come up and speak on his supernatural healing. But as this vision turned to dust and I would never have the chance to see if this miracle working power would materialize in his life. As I felt this decision should not have rested with this person, as my brother was God's man unequally yoked and would have given another a chance to at least see if the body would heal. Although the law provides over 45 days, and I wanted to give my brother a chance to live and even offered to have him moved to another facility to no avail. But the hospital did not listen or value anyone else's opinion and his wife ignored me. This puts to rest the mystery of why there are more single people today than ever before in history. I was devastated as well as my son, and left my home of over ten years overnight, as I had to just do something to try to cope. I also asked my oldest brother to help as he took his younger brother's passing just as hard. I stayed on my feet for days packing, unpacking, and moving boxes. My feet stayed swollen and in between the moving, I shed tears and reminisced on everything. Reminiscing on his extraordinary ingenious childhood to his forever giving adulthood, as everyone who knew him loved him. He raised numerous children, two of his own and all who knew him loved him dearly. My brother was even about to help me build a getaway house in the country.

We were not only hurt but angry, and I had to continually keep uplifting God especially before my son, as I did not want him to loose his faith. I had seen in my life God's miracle working power as I was able to pray for my brother's healing as he had lost his mind before to some bad drugs during his teenage years. So I had to continue on for those of us who are still here.

I guess after knowing and loving a person your entire life and not having a say so in what may or may not be the final days of their life is most disturbing. It is an event you never get over, but you just learn to live with the pain as best you can. This was most devastating as I could not even listen to any music or even sit trying to live normally, as my laughter would eventually end up with gut wrenching tears. Immediately afterwards I would hear testimony after testimony from people being healed after weeks on life support, and the doctors had given up hope. They all talked of how their entire families had faith and prayed and did not give up hope and within weeks, they were waking up with their bodies recovering.

Although I cannot blame myself, I can maybe try to help someone else by telling my story. As I had previously struggled to heal my mother and now my brother is gone, I could not forget all the strides that have been made in the medical field. Strides such as early detection of blocked arteries and other diseases. Our American as well as African American doctors and other pioneers made great contributions to the medical field, and more specifically in the field of heart surgery would no doubt be flabbergasted to learn how many Americans and more specifically African American lives are shortened unnecessarily by untreated circulatory conditions.

Today, our medical community is in fact deciding who lives and who dies and the so called underdog of the society is not receiving adequate nutrition and medical care. Being deprived of fair and adequate medical assistance as far as new and life saving procedures and technologies, that are offered as normal practice for certain hospitals. This is not fair and must be addressed by our federal government in the proper manner whether than trying to institute monetary limit in lawsuits. We need to set federal guidelines that all hospitals must follow based on the medical technology and treatment that should and must be made available to all patients. There must be some laws passed to address these issues if society does not want to continue to pay for these mistakes via the court's time and money.

One example of life saving technologies not traditionally offered for regular or the so called "under class" include liver transplants. A portion of the liver from a healthy relative or other donor can be transplanted to the person who needs a liver. Subsequently, both the donor and donee with proper nutrition can in fact rebuild the liver back to normal functionality. This is just one example of what could be offered as a normal procedure or option for the patient, and followed routinely just as other needed procedures for conditions considered life threatening or eventual life threatening illness required to save a life. In short, this country should be saving its citizens lives no matter what one's class, creed, color, or background may be. We have the technology and now we are trying to play God in deciding who lives and who does not. If we have the knowhow, we should save all lives we will receive in return what we give in this life and I would much rather help people and give life as this produces no regrets. Medical treatment and nutrition should go hand and hand and in some cases our medical community has somehow become confused and is not committed to all humanity. But certain individuals in the medical community are continually making uninformed, or just plain ill-fated decisions in respect to the average or underclass in respect to who should live and who should not. The underclass I am referring to are persons like myself and my brother and mother who are good hard working people in this society and have practically given their entire life to this country by their hard work and love for their fellow man. Sometimes overlooking their own health and safety to save another. My brother was a child prodigy, an unknown genius whom acquired most of his smarts from my ingenious mother who graduated number one from Phyllis Wheatley High School. As Texas Southern University pleaded with my brother to apply as he had scored the highest ever on the GED taken there, as he was bored with high school. His high school teachers, as well as his elementary teachers marveled at his brilliance, but could not keep him challenged in his classes. As we were all born from meager means and my brother was finally left at a point in his life as the great Langhston Huges would define "a dream deferred".

So now my prayer continues on, and "I pray that may our God in heaven help us to love one another no matter what our status in this life may appear to be".

I have a beautiful picture my brother Charles drew and sent to me on February 2nd 2004 not long after my mother passed in December 2003. I happened to keep it, and now it is most precious to me as it portrays the lettering of my name with a cross along with a bible verse.

Little did I know at the time that this verse would serve to be some form of comfort in this most disastrous time.  As it reads: ***"What shall we then say to these things? If God is for us, then who can be against us?" Romans 8:31***

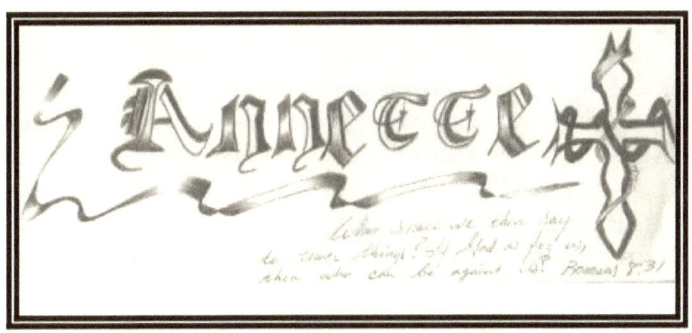

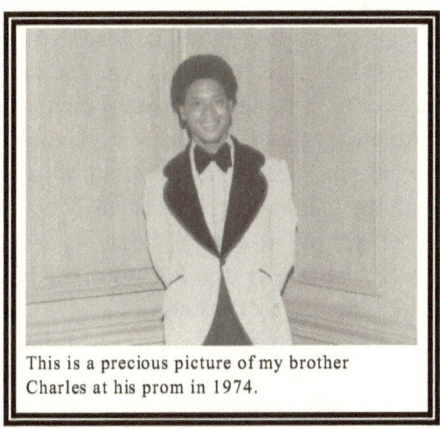

This is a precious picture of my brother Charles at his prom in 1974.

*"I have come to heal the brokenhearted...........to set at liberty those that are bruised"* .

*St Luke*

Chapter 8: Conclusion:  A PHILOSOPHICAL VIEW ON LIFE TODAY:
*'BECOMING A WHOLE PERSON, MIND BODY AND SOUL'*

Today as I try to live my life as a relatively whole person after all the mistakes and unhappy situations, I continue to strive toward excellence while constantly pondering the past for reasons and answers. Answers to why so many mistakes as well as questioning the reasons of how and why I am here?  Will I continue to make mistakes or have I come to a place in my life of comfort and peace?

As most I have even endeavored to question the very existence of this great world. The true history of this great country reveals sometimes very mixed feelings.  Although I love life just as many others yet in the mist of feelings of joy, the sorrow and even sometimes feelings of disarray develop.

In the past I have sometimes felt as though two very different people are pulling and tugging in my very soul, but yet they exist and live quite comfortably inside my mind.  On the far right deep inside the very debts of my soul I feel the horrors and pain of the slave taken into captivity, and literally wiped from their very existence.  Literally wiped from one's own mother, father, and other siblings or cousins, aunts, uncles, grandparents, and beyond.  The family that held all the purpose and meaning is left behind in Africa which was a most fatal blow, that will be ingrained in the family tree for hundreds of years to come.  No one person could escape the devastating pain.  Thus, can the pain become greater, for those who survive?  Yes indeed I think it can, but for those who attempted to continue a meaningful existence thrived on the love.  Love of those who survived became a close nit family of slaves.  These persons of course not enjoying the slavery, but sought refuge in their families.  The family was the only thing that kept them at peace and with any shred of dignity.  Then unexpectedly and very tragically, the horrid nightmare continued to unfold as slave owners faced financial hardships.  Some slaves were once again sold like merchandise to the highest bidder and torn away from their families in America.  As more human sacrifices of pain instilled more anguish in a people we now call today, Americans.

How can we bare the pain from Mother Africa and the shame of Europe and still live without experiencing flashbacks ingrained in our souls. For my heritage reveals that of an African American woman and a French man. I feel her ancestry pain and I feel his unrenowned anguish. They both reside in me although I did not know this African woman nor did I know this French man. And after all the history of pain, I do know I love my life this day. For certain, I did not always feel this way, as my heart appeared to mask much of this ingrained pain.

Sometimes I feel as though the anger and abuse from my ancestors inhabited the very existence of my soul, and though I try to forgo the pain it surfaces again. On one hand I was a proud American, and yet also feeling some shame and degradation. So we choose to live the proud lie while subconsciously continuing to feel like our ancestors. Some of our ancestors wished to die while trying and sometimes succeeding at killing their newborn children. This ancestry pain or curse passed down for generations, as it manifested itself through my repeated mistakes. Other persons may have experienced the exact same ancestry pain, or it may have been very different more of a slow and silent subconscious killer. Mentally fighting and rebelling against everything you were taught and know in your heart is right, while havoc reeks in one's life choices. Sometimes surfacing through drug abuse, depression, eating disorders, continued economical dysfunctions, aborting a fetus, or even worst murder of human being in cold blood. It is like a heedless wound passed from generation to generation. I would be born into a world facing a curse of misfortune that I would ultimately have to overcome or it would destroy me just as has destroyed millions of others.

I just like many others had to grasp the true fact, that I did not love what I was doing or myself. Hence, this created a constant battlefield within me. Although at times I felt like I was the most beautiful person in the world, there were other times I felt like the most dismal person alive. Mainly during my failed relationships, I blamed my unhappiness on others and hated my life. Every thing that was not perfect took residence in my soul, and it would ultimately dictate the negative order of my life. Within the very depths of my soul resounded a silent unrelenting death wish. Some desire to die out of honor, while I would just merely want to die without truly understanding the real reasons why.  If I had not realized where and how this self-inflicting pain materialized in my life I would have destroyed myself for reasons never really known to me, or others like me.  This was nothing short of a haunting curse from the pass that I had to breakthrough.  I had to breakthrough all the ideas of right and wrong, of a history of pain, of hatred and self-loathing, and fill this void with love.  As my parents instilled in me compassion and love for others, I still needed to embrace self-love.

The key to embracing self love is to finally look at myself without thinking of all the negative connotations.  This included removing all the degrading references such as all the "n" words.  The small but most powerful words in reference an African American to make one feel somewhat less of a human being.

I had to put to rest all the physical negatives that may unknowingly haunt the psychic as one may refer to an African American or as an African American may refer to another.  The first physical negative I had to dispel was referring to  hair as nappy.  I figured out that anyone's hair can be tangled after you wet it or wash it with bar soap.  As most African Americans did not have the luxury or natural herbal ingredients readily available that mostly originated from the Motherland to make the hair more manageable.  This is what we now very commonly refer to as 'detangling shampoos' and 'conditioners'.  Items that not only make the hair more manageable, but also give a luster and beauty that our American ancestors would eventually and slowly recognize as they were given the opportunity tap into their own creative abilities.  Hence, I replaced that "n" word with "fluffy".  Fluffy hair became a much more precise and accurate term as even Jesus had fluffy hair like lambs wool, so it was no less than beautiful.  The word 'Negro', was definitely unacceptable and I did not care for it, as this term was too much like the other "n" word that I chose not to spell out, which was derived during a time of deep routed prejudice and it signifies an evil profanity to me.

Self-loathing was causing me to continually reek havoc in my life, which manifested itself into feelings of insecurity.  My childhood molestation lingered in my mind, while I attempted to block it out as best I could.  My adult rapes added more havoc and helped to solidify repeated pregnancies after the birth of my son, and his father absence. These events would materialize into giving me a legitimate way to judge true love, which was most inappropriate and mostly unreasonable. Finally I decided I could not let the pass control my future.  I had to leave all the negative shames behind, and let God with his never-ending mercy console me, as it was my only relief.  As I look back on my life before the birth of my son, I could have avoided a lot of my dilemma's if I had at least taken some professional karate classes.  But as far as my life after the birth of my son, although I was able to reconcile within myself and deal with most of the mistakes from the past, the issue of aborting a fetus was still most difficult.  This issue was like any other addiction. Unconsciously continuing the same mind set by surrounding myself with the same type of acquaintances tends to give rise to an addiction, while simply fooling myself into thinking I could exhibit perseverance.

Whether we are engaging in uninhibited premarital bliss, aborting unborn fetuses, merely eating inappropriately resulting in an unhealthy body, continuing to smoke and doing drugs, or even stealing or even hurting another, this is all in fact lashing out at one's inner self. It is no doubt self-hatred that drives us to our most morbid actions.

By taking birth control pills we not only inhibit the development of the fetus by altering the woman's natural ability to ovulate, but create a greater risk of developing life-threatening illness.  The risk of cancer, stroke, heart attack, obesity, and other health problems and disease that can ultimately lead to death.  I further feel very strongly that I would have been one of those few that the possible risks would have materialized in.  Maybe it was God leading me as well as taking care of me in the mist of my sometimes ill-fated circumstances.

As I try to reason and make sense of my actions, in terms of all the abortions after the birth of my son , which some would term just plain subverted and irrational behavior.  Although there was basically not any reasonable justification, most of the time I felt like why take the pill when I do not believe in engaging in premarital bliss.  But as I would continue to meet people and hormones continued to rage, and in some cases I eventually developed relationships and would end up compromising my beliefs. The birth control pill always made me ill and I often experienced severe headaches, and inevitably I would stop taking them. I would often times just discontinue the pill just to feel better. More often than not my companion did not like using a condom for protection, which would lead me to conclude most of the unplanned pregnancies were not even all my fault.

I went even further with my need to find some justification in this abortion dilemma. As I attempted to evaluate the analogy of right and wrong in the context of choosing the option of birth control in the form of pills versus an abortion. While I do not condone abortion as a means of birth control, I had to analyze it in the context of what does 'right' truly mean. As most of the abortion activist may view abortion as morally wrong, they may accept birth control pills or condoms as the right thing to do. Consider if one opts to use some form of birth control, one is still no doubt altering the body's natural effects of nature by inhibiting the development of an unborn fetus. So if we really want to consider this issue as a matter of right and wrong, one should quite possibly not even consider engaging in the act without considering the possibility of conception. As I feel most often making love is reduced to an act of mere lust, which is just as wrong as abortion. Hence, one can conclude whether abortion or taking birth control pills, one is still prohibiting the development of a fetus and ultimately the birth of a child. Both of these concepts can be considered the same in the context of right and wrong. I feel that in fact the birth control pill just as abortion, are the exact same in theory as they inhibit the birth of a fetus.

As I regret my actions, I feel they were very much unavoidable. Although I could never abandon or destroy a child I would have given birth to, I did choose to abort a fetus. A fetus that one of the parents did not want, and I could never bring another into the world that would not receive the love he or she deserved. Although my son's father had major issues and was not involved in his life as needed, I do feel he loved his son. I had the love of both my parents and could not imagine life any other way.

Although I have always felt making love should occur after marriage, I further feel not just because of the AIDS epidemic which is most definitely reason enough, that everyone should practice safe sex by using condoms. This poses the least amount of medical risks and mental dilemma's. Medical risks in terms of the warning signs leading to unwarranted ailments and possibly contacting a major disease from taking birth control pills. Also, the possibility of contacting further disease or infection from the unprotected act itself. Some individuals may have a mental dilemma from being forced or coerced into the act itself, as I was. Also from taking a chance by not using any protection and later suffering mental anguish by opting to have an abortion; as I exhibited some risk factors and sometimes chose to stop taking pills. I was prone to certain diseases as I exhibited symptoms, in which the risk increases with the pill. Hence, condoms ultimately can create a safer environment for both individuals physical well being without altering the female's natural body cycles.

Furthermore, lust and love are not the same and are two very opposite and different feelings that can be quite confusing. The only way to distinguish between the two involves not engaging in the act of making love unless you can see yourself having a child or a family with the person, and until you are mentally and financially ready for the responsibility of children one should always practice safe sex or abstain. As a society there are instances where we may have the tendency to reduce the act of making love, which entails two people in love, into a lustful act of just merely sex to satisfy hormonal urges. Also, a past taboo was placed on lovemaking, as most of my role models from mom to minister avoided discussing the topic details.


During one of the occurrences of reconciling myself to God, I had a brief meeting with a minister. It was a rather brief friendship, but for some reason I exposed a bit of my pass. He also exposed very personal details of how his son was born out of wedlock. He further diagnosed my current situation as being unable to move pass the failed relationship with my son's father. I had not come to grips with the reality that although I had a beautiful son, and his father, for whatever reasons was not apart of our lives. In short this minister concluded, "You need to move on with life in a positive manner while forgiving Joseph's father for his shortcomings." As he continued in a mostly soft but very saddened voice, "Your negative relationship experience is holding you back from experiencing a wonderful life with another. It has been over ten years and you have to let go." He concluded I held a lot of anger and pain within me, which could only be released by forgiving my son's father. It was no doubt a reality that some of my actions, in these subsequent relationships to follow would mask this truth. I guess in the back of my mind the thought of Joe and I getting back together was always there, and that thought contributed to the decisions I made in my life. Also, I felt an unquestionable sense of distrust for men and it too was holding me back as well. I further needed to love myself no matter how many mistakes I had made, I needed to realize I was worth something and I did not necessarily need anyone else to validate my existence as a complete and fulfilled person.

I finally realized in the absence of my son's father the role I played out in these unwarranted pregnancies after my son's father left may have also been a subconscious attempt to legitimize, or rather give me a reason to move pass this relationship and go on with my life. As I wanted so to be able to give my son the father figure he deserved and the family I yearned for, but I did not actually trust or want to move on with my life with another. Not only was I going about it wrong and in a mostly unenlightened way, but also I was neglecting my inner joy and peace in the process. So maybe I would not actually free myself from my continued mistakes until I forgave Joseph's father and put to rest any type of future life with this man.

The only thing I did know for certain was that I needed closure, so I sat down and wrote a letter. I told him how I didn't really know if it mattered to him, but I needed to tell him I forgave him. I had been holding on to these bad feelings and I felt the only way to move on was to write him. I further wished him joy, peace, happiness as well as the hope he would one day straighten out his life. In so much as Joseph was a teenager and appeared to no longer look for that father figure, I still felt he needed someone to talk to. As I continued to try dating once again looking for the right person that Joseph would be able to confide in, I ended up once again with disappointment. As I decided to just raise and protect my son while caring for my mother as best I could. As Jonathan saved my life and gave me a reason to live, and my mother needed me in a different but similar capacity. These were the responsibilities in my life that gave me a fulfilled life.

We must understand that no matter how much pain fills our pass, one must rise above it and continue to focus on the dream that will ultimately materialize into our prosperous future. One must continue to focus on the end results, your dream, no matter what your present circumstances may be. If I had dwelled on being poor and economically disadvantaged, molestation's, bad decisions, I would have never gave a thought to attending college much less returning time after time until I reached my goal. One must continue to look pass the negative past that we did not even have a choice in the matter, while understanding we all may make some mistakes that we are not particularly proud of. For somewhere deep inside all of us resides that persistent person, who never gives up, as I do believe one person can change the world. By learning and educating ourselves about our family history, this country, as well as the history of the world one can move ahead. If I had not moved pass the mistakes, the anger, the self-hatred, and the shame of pass injustices it would inevitably eliminated me as a person as well as my need to aspire and create.

Today I have come to the realization that I am first and foremost an American. And although I am not my ancestors nor my parents, I am a whole new and different person, I must further recognize all these virtues of my past has no doubt made me what I am today. All the past choices from my ancestors to my parents help shape me into what I am today. But now I am a person, not like any other in the world but very alike in many ways. Americans though very different from any other culture in the world, in that we search freely and have the choice to find and dictate our future. Yet we are all very much alike in that all cultures search for the true meaning of this thing we call life.

I truly believe mankind's desire to fulfill basic instincts tend to cause setbacks in our ability to achieve and accomplish, as we mistakenly substitute immediate needs for true self-fulfillment. For example, if we hunger we fulfill that desire with whatever may taste or just look good. We never think about what we are eating, but rather we are strictly functioning based on our instincts. We further have diminished love making to merely an act of necessity, rather than the beautiful and wondrous ultimate display of love. Hence, one must rise above this animal instinct in order to achieve. The psyche or brain must be nourished physically by proper nutrition and developed mentally through education, in order for one to make logical choices in life. Then we are able to contribute to making this world better through creating, building and expounding technologies, which leads to innovative scientific achievements. This is our true and natural human instinct. If we are created in the image of God, then we must act as Gods rising above animal instinct or any pattern of behavior that would in fact destroy our creative abilities which is a most needed fate.

So whatever the negative shames one might experience in their life, how does one move to a higher plain and another does not. The answer lies in one owns self worth. Although my parents instilled self-confidence as well as the love of God in my life, I still had to work through my own varied and mixed feelings and the true meaning of life for myself. But through perseverance and prayer, I managed to tap back into that greatness of life I felt as a young child. Prayer not only corrects the pass mistakes of mankind, but it helps to release our own feelings of guilt. I have reached a very different plain or level in life, thereby releasing myself from all the pain of the past that I created for myself. Furthermore, one must have some kind of positive influence in their life. I do believe this is the only way one moves out of shame and into the prosperity of a successful life. After I sometimes lived my confused life in resistance to everything my parents taught about God, I always ended up back praying to God for help time after time. Afterwards life appeared much clearer, it was truly easier to just do the right thing. I finally came to the realization that God was indeed real and I needed his saving grace in my life continually, or I would quite possibly continue to fail.  For far too long I based my life on the very negative tragedies that gave rise to the physical instincts, while neglecting my intellectual development.  I had to move back to square one and began the chest game once more, and this time I desired to win.


        Throughout my life I truly felt God was ordering my steps, or else I might not be the person I am today.  As I looked back over my life this time in order to begin once again, the first thing I recall would be my father dying of a fatal heart attack.  Not long afterwards during my childhood I decided to become a doctor to try to make a difference, as this
started to give me a sense of my self worth. He developed heart disease before I would start grade school.  My cousin also left us prematurely from heart problems as well as a host of relatives, whom left this world due to hardening of the arteries, brain disorders, infection, and other types of disease.  Their life span cut far too short due to very different but also quite similar tragedies.  But when my Mother was slowly leaving me in 1996, I knew if I just called on the name of Jesus that something had to happen.  So, I made the most life altering and important decision I would probably ever make and would ever make again, as I decided to become the primary caregiver for my aging and ailing mother.  My Mother suffering from a previous diagnosis of diverticulitis, rheumatoid arthritis which caused her to stop walking, high blood pressure, circulatory problems, and lastly the congestive heart failure as I just continued to pray.
        As I prayed I attempted to acquire some reasonable knowledge by reading everything I could about the conditions of my mother's diagnosis.  Thus gaining knowledge on these situations made me feel more in control of my life.  Now I would finally begin to feel peace as I gained knowledge.  Knowledge is in fact power as I began to see my feelings of insecurity dwindle to faint images of a broken, and yet meaningful pass.  Although I still quench at the thoughts of some of the horrible mistakes of my pass, I can't help but feel the pass may have contributed to the place I am today.  A person of compassion, unrelenting

hope, and determination.  As I chose the responsibility of primary caregiver for my mother, I do feel and will always feel I made a crucial decision that could not change my grim pass,  but might enable a more fulfilling future.

In the mist of my tears and prayers I heard a still soft voice in my spirit saying , everything is alright.  As I felt a sense of guilt from the circumstances of this world began to lift from my weary shoulders, and it was as though I had finally transferred all my burdens to God himself.  I have further come to the realization that probably this quest for knowledge only began, because my mother was unable to care for herself.  As my mother's eventual passing took place while at home, I know beyond a reasonable doubt if I had been with her she would not have passed that day.  But I also know that I needed help and could not have cared for her alone, and further had to accept that I did the very best I could.

I cannot change any of grim past and unhealthy living, but now I do still hold the key to fulfilling the future.  I can at least try to continue to break this generational curse of sickness and disease.  Now I just try to help anyone who is willing to listen, from giving family members good food and vitamins as gift baskets as well as talking to coworkers to strangers about the importance of good dietary habits.

As I look at some immediate family members continuing to overindulge, while I attempted to make my mother's pain go away.  I watch us continuing toward the horror of never ending pain, I watch in sorrow as we drink and eat too much of all the wrong foods and neglect our health.  We cannot simply continue to ignore the fact Helen's condition or any other health problem does not just happen, but there are causes and effects in every aspect of our lives.  We must take responsibility by either obtaining the proper test and diagnosis from our health professionals to eating nutritionally sound foods, to exercising which includes weight training and stretching.  This may ultimately be some of the key differences between caring for ourselves, or others caring for us.  This general premise not only applies to the aging but as certain food continues to be mass-produced with preservatives such as hydrogenated oils along with the possibility of some of our food becoming polluted with mercury and other chemicals, this becomes a harsh reality for young people as well. But through my knowledge and research I continue to pray and believe we can break the curse of early death in our family and other families as well, as we may all be able to age gracefully while reminiscing upon the good old days as we sip a good cup of herbal tea.

In my not so distant past I never had any desire to drink tea, as my preference was soda. Now I drink tea upon arising, sometimes throughout the day, and even before bedtime. This lifestyle change was definitely nothing short of a miracle. Not only have I expounded on some of the positive teachings from my parents as a child, but I have exposed myself to other wonderful teachings as well. I have been able to integrate both worlds and make tremendous growth. I could not make a change without first regaining my metal ability to think logically. Not just eliminating the unwarranted chemicals such as medications, but also changes in my diet and exercise helped me become a whole person again.

It is further important that we listen to our bodies and become aware of warning signs. We must try to eliminate any risk factors that could contribute to sickness and disease not only to our body, but our mind as well.

As I have found some people are born with certain innate physical characteristics. In other words you will look like your mother, father, or some other relative or ancestor. You will further carry or exhibit their traits, such as thick hair, freckled skin, and even a weak or a strong immune system. It can further be characterized in even carrying a trait or gene for alcoholism. These are your genetic characteristics and can be beneficial or detrimental to the very nature of your life. In other words one could live a very healthy life or unhealthy life based on a predetermined genetic background, which can be defined as risk factors. But there are other underlying risk factors such as nutritional characteristics or deficiencies to consider in our daily lives as well. These are the risk factors that can and will help us either maintain our beneficial traits or exploit our detrimental hereditary traits.

Let us look at the traits of a person who is born with a healthy bone structure and as they age a deteriorating bone disease sets in, or a person without any history of high blood pressure or heart disease but develops the chronic condition. Even though some conditions may be hereditary, the other primary reason why we need to look at family history is because if your father ate certain foods or smoked and developed a chronic heart condition, then more often than not you will eat the same foods and end up with the same chronic condition as well. But more importantly we must consider the general dietary habits of this individual over time, and ask how it played a role or how we can overcome the factors of genetic ailments. More often than not it is a nutritional relationship rather than just a hereditary factor.

Further nutritional risk factors develop over time, for example, one person who smokes the same number of cigarettes daily does not develop cancer or heart disease until forty years of smoking, whereas another may develop heart disease within twenty years. Or take for instance an elderly person who develops Alzheimer's disease and one who does not. Dietary differences may play a significant role in each of these scenarios. We may conclude this may be no doubt a miracle, but also there may be dietary differences. One person may be consuming adequate daily amounts antioxidants such as vitamin "E" and "low acidic C", foods rich in B Complex more specifically B-12, or other dietary considerations such as zinc. In other words we need to look at what we may be doing differently such as the foods we are consuming, as well as know their nutritional value. Although this scenario may not answer all of our health questions, it could probably be a good start for answering some of these complex questions of illness. I am not by any means saying that one should go out and smoke and if you take supplements you will not develop disease over time, because some supplements such as beta carotene and drinking alcohol have been shown to create an even more adverse environment for the liver of a drinker, etc. But what I am saying is proper nutrition can protect the body over time from certain ailments. Also there can be nutritional related treatments such as certain components in soy that can in fact aid in overcoming deficiencies and ailments related to possible hereditary conditions, such as alcoholism susceptibility or other weaknesses such as hormone imbalance. Additionally other hereditary ailments or hormone related imbalances such as Cushing that if identified can be treated appropriately, staph infections treated more expeditiously, or contagious conditions such as H. pylori bacteria can be treated with various antibiotics and monitored with repeated breath tests until completely healed.

Hence, there are several varying reasons why the human body becomes sick or ill, and there can be several ways to treat and eventually achieve a healthy environment in the body.

One cannot even think rationally when polluting the body with bad foods, water, or chemicals that can create a toxic state in the human body. As I recall my sad yet unchanging past mistakes and sometimes wonder how I could make such irresponsible choices. But further recall my inappropriate dietary habits, and how everything I knew was best ended up being overshadowed by the inability to logically reason. I just acted and reacted to situations, never logically thinking through the situation prior to acting. Not only did I fail to eat right but abused medications, which further inhibited my ability to think rationally. As I can attribute all my illogical actions, including my raging hormones to improper diet. Although I am not making any excuses for my choices in life, your diet can either help your health or be detrimental to your health and this includes every part of the human body as well as the mind's thought process. I have further found that certain foods including plants, herbs, seeds, and nuts have a medicinal and positive effect on the body. On the other hand chemicals from preservatives and certain medications and inappropriate eating can be very serious and toxic to the human body. This causes negative affects and can damage any organ in the body including the brain, which I term as the very heart and soul of the human body. Without a sound mind one cannot function or do anything constructive for yourself or anyone else.

Although I feel my mother cooked mostly nutritious meals for the family, there were a few dietary concerns due to some aspect of our diet. My mother cooked mostly beans, rice, cornbread, and greens which was unknown to me and probably my whole family at time a complete protein and most nutritious meal. But I was a very finicky eater and did not want any part of the meal, and due to my diet from childhood into my young adulthood, I stayed sick. I had colds and flu every year, kidney as well as other infections, and an appendectomy as a teenager. As a child I recall my mother keeping either a can of lard or an aluminum pan of leftover lard. We further had a can that actually said 'G R E A SE' vertically down the front of the can, which included a strainer that we used for everything from used lard to straining leftover bacon drippings. This was stored daily not only to conserve as we were considered financially challenged, but for seasoning as it was added to just about every meal.

Even into my adulthood the colds and flu continued, and I would get so sick I would be bed bound for at least a week. After I had my son by cesarean I further developed fibroid tumors, which pushed on my rectum and bladder. So I finally had the benign tumors removed, only for them to return in a few months. Between the medications and having surgeries to correct the problems, it merely masked the situations and never really corrected the root cause. The root cause being my dietary habits as I ate lots of meat and foods treated with hormones and added artificial properties. This resulted in a hormone imbalance which help contribute to the fibroid tumors. Additionally, I had a deviated septum, TMJ problems in my jaw, and even a small benign knot on he back of my neck from a car accident. As I have further had several other surgical procedures, some of which included bad root canals resulting in tooth removals. I felt the root canals probably were due to the enlarged fillings, which might have been done unnecessarily during my childhood. These were all no doubt some of my risk factors that contributed to my unhealthy lifestyle.

Other risk factors that contribute to illness and disease include excess salt, too much sugar, and eating too many noncomplex carbohydrates such man made fortified grains. Eating fiber based complex carbohydrates such as whole grains, and lots fruits and vegetables help keep the body regulated which starts with the digestive track and transcends to a whole healthy body. Also cultured foods such as tofu, yogurt, mushrooms, and other foods as well as supplements that contribute to good intestinal flora. Non-complex carbohydrates such as white flour, white bread, sweet rolls and other pastries contain no germ or rather no essential fiber. Although these altered grains may be fortified with vitamins such as folate, niacin, calcium, iron, etc., these vitamins can be received from your food and a good whole food vitamin supplement. Other complex carbs include whole grain bread and pasta, cereal such as kashi, some fresh popped popcorn with a little olive oil, brown rice, quinoa, and amaranth. Flaxseed as well as walnuts contains essential omega fatty acids.

Eating lots of animal products such as red meat, dairy products, and other saturated fats such as hydrogenated oils including palm and coconut oils contribute to elevated cholesterol levels. Whole grains, seeds, and natural nuts without any added preservatives are vital to help prevent sickness and disease such as stroke, heart attack, etc. The most ideal scenario is leaving the grains whole rather than removing naturally occurring nutrients, adding unwarranted hydrogenated oils, bleaching agents, and preservatives resulting in chemically treated foods which all create health risks. These procedures became the norm in the early to mid 1900's and so came the additional health problems. It appears to me more economical to produce the food as is, instead of spending money on altering the structural content. The most important way to prevent risk factors is through proper diet. Eating right and taking a good whole food multiple vitamins can ease our cravings for sweets, carbohydrates, and other such foods that can cause health risks. Eating a well-balanced and proportioned meal remains vitally important and cannot be taken lightly. It is no joke, as I had to continually monitor my ailing mother's condition. You can either sacrifice now by eating right and exercising, or pay later. As I watched family members and even my mother's condition worsen throughout my childhood, I can unequivocally state proper diet as well as exercise and sunlight should not be taken lightly.

A healthy lifestyle should be the center of our very existence coming in second to nothing, because how can one have a meaningful life if you cannot function properly either physically or mentally. After my needed dietary changes, I began to have a different and a more positive view on life. It was as though the same little girl who sat in the swing over thirty years ago dreaming had resurfaced once again. I can only pray I keep my same outlook, as I desire so deeply to practice this lifestyle. As we cannot predict our life span, we can at practice a healthy existence as we continue to age.

The most crucial yet inevitable fact reveals if we want to have a healthy mind and body we must in fact be proactive by educating ourselves. Not relying on others for knowledge, while still not totally eliminating our family physician for our well-being. We have to renew our minds taking full control and responsibility for our circumstances. Not to wallow in misery or feel sorry for ourselves, but realizing there is a cause and effect. Nothing just happens, and no matter what age, family background, or economic status we must start today to achieve goals in life while reaching and striving for that higher plain. I am living prove that one can start this day, because I am forty something and an aspiring pre-med student.

I had a choice to do the right thing not just for a few days, but rather a change in my entire way of living, a lifestyle change. Leaving all the past shames behind and not look at life the same way, but having a renewed and refreshed zest for life.

This lifestyle change not only includes dietary changes but vigorously exercising daily, which help cleanse the body, which ultimately produces an attitude change. In other words exercise results in a total healthy body, which includes a healthy brain as your circulation increases the oxygen flow to the brain. One must exercise vigorously such as aerobics or jogging at least ten to twenty minutes daily or three times a week for thirty to forty minutes, which brings the heart rate up while strengthening the heart muscle. Increasing the heart rate is the ideal scenario for a healthy body. Sweating helps eliminate toxins through the largest organ in our bodies, which is the skin. Besides cleansing our bodies through proper diet and fasting, toxins can be released through the skin. Once a lifestyle change has been achieved, one can inevitably look toward a renewed mind, body, and soul.

Although I feel no one person in the human race can cure all types of illnesses, we can definitely avoid most of it through proper dietary habits, exercise, and by exhibiting some self control. Self-control is no doubt the most difficult, but one must always keep the following two rules in mind.

First and foremost, I removed items from my home and discontinued purchasing the food items that cause a most unhealthy environment such as candy, sodas, chips, white bread, or any non-nutritious food item. Replaced those items with a *high fiber* regiment including at least 80% fresh fruits and vegetables, whole grains such as high fiber oats and wheat germ, and also needed protein to maintain a healthy body. The only way to actively and naturally remove or lower the bad cholesterol in my diet is through a high fiber regiment. A complete vegetarian protein substitute equals beans including split peas, whole grain rice such as quinoa or brown rice, and corn. Other high protein items such as veggie-burgers or tofu, a whole food natural protein drink, and other nutritious foods that I want to include along with the herbal seasonings mentioned in the previous chapters. A natural whole food vegetable protein drink with sea vegetables such as spirulina and chlorella, kelp, alfalfa, rice bran, royal jelly, FOS such as acidophilus provide healthy intestinal bacteria, and other great ingredients are a better choice for providing your complete protein (all amino acids) rather than taking them separately. More importantly some sea vegetables along with other vital nutrients such as vitamin C, etc, also appear to assist in weight management. Including yogurt with the protein drink also helps maintain digestion as it contains acidophilus. Eating fresh fruits in the morning such as grapefruit and apples and other fresh fruits and vegetables before my protein, as they contain digestive enzymes to help break down food. Also, hormone and enzyme activity decrease with age, because it is continually used not only to digest food but for every single body action, such as movement and healing functions. Enzymes are needed to digest your food and vital vitamins and minerals consumed daily. Life cannot be sustained without proper digestion, as your cells will not be able survive without acquiring or absorbing the needed nutrients.

In my case which is similar to most aging adults I needed to add some natural supplements. Most importantly I sometimes added garlic along with a vegetarian pancreatic proteolytic enzyme formula to help breakdown my foods and proteins, and help control my reoccurring tumors along with maintaining a proper diet.  I added other supplements mentioned previously such as B-complex vitamins for proper system balance including B-12 ( for proper nerve function), folic acid, niacin as well as biotin a hair nutrient that help break down proteins, choline and L-Carnitine (an amino acid) that are brain nutrients that help metabolize fat and are considered good fat burners.  But basically, I do not recommend taking your amino acids separately as they have a synergy affect and we need to take our proteins in there complete form for proper nutrition and health.  But I do occasionally take carnitine and/or lysine also found in corn (an essential amino acid for calcium and collagen absorption, tissue/muscle repair, and proper balance).  Also including the mineral magnesium, and sometimes an amino acid, L-methionine, which both help prevent fat buildup in the arteries.  I later learned after caring for my deceased mother and the unwarranted demise of my brother, that fermented soybean called "nattokinase" has been shown to help decrease fibrinogen build up.  And further learned some concentrated species of brown seaweed formulas are showing great promise in everything from detoxification to circulatory conditions to cancer.

Additionally, including rice, oat or almond milk and yogurt for needed calcium.  Calcium rich foods help maintain the system alkaline balance as an over acidic system can cause various diseases.

Cauliflower is further considered a brain nutrient as it contains choline, one of the b-complex essential brain nutrients.  Choline is also a prime ingredient in some diets, as I had excellent results taking Choline with L-Carnitine and sometimes including a little caffeine. Mushrooms are also showing great promise in building my immune system. Specifically, shitake , miatake and reishi or red mushrooms can assist in immune system response to fight off contaminates in my body. Cauliflower, broccoli, brussel sprouts, and kale are considered cruciferous vegetables, which are excellent for colon health and even help fight abnormal cell growth which includes cancer. Antioxidants such as vitamin E are also good for the brain, heart nutrient CoQ10, fish oils rich in omega 3, a non acidic vitamin C, all assist with proper cell functions and system balance, as well as high fiber foods and fiber

supplements. The normal recommended dosage of fiber should at least
be thirty milligrams a day.

Also I include my gingko tea with other brain nutrients such as
lemon grass, celery seed, sage, and other herbs, as well as sometimes
including an aspirin to help protect the brain and circulatory system.

Being  creative with my meals such as melting vege-cheese on
leftover turkey or all natural turkey slices with sprouts, green-mix lettuce
leaves, garlic, onions, apples, mushrooms, while sprinkling granulated
kelp for seasoning to help maintain an alkaline system. Kelp or other
seaweed can be used in place of salt but is also available in liquid and
capsule form, I sometimes take it in some of my vegetarian protein
powders as most good protein powders will have added brown seaweed
such as kelp.  But all brown seaweed contains vital minerals and supports
my brain, nerves, nails, blood vessels, hair, obesity, ulcers, and protects
against radiation. If I have to use salt I use only sea salt.  Make an
organic salad with fresh celery, onions, garlic, mustard, cauliflower or
broccoli, vegetarian meat, and a little organic honey and lemon juice
with a whole grain spouted tortilla or pita.  Beets or sometimes
cucumbers make great snacks while adding a little sea salt and kelp for a
tastier snack.  I always try to eat a small portion of fresh fruit before my
meal and fresh vegetables with the meal. You will soon find that your
taste buds and body love these fresh fruits and vegetables filled with
nutrients, as well as much needed water.  The body requires at least 64
ounces of purified water daily to maintain a cognitive and clear mind, a
good outlook on life, and firm muscles.  Also I tested the ph balance of
my water as well as my body for a too acidic or alkaline system by
ordering some ph paper from the pharmacy. Then I started adding foods
that help balance my body by adding alkaline foods, in order to eliminate
an overly acidic environment.  As previously mentioned acidic foods
include all foods with added sugar such as junk foods and sodas, meats,
coffee, tea, cocoa, pepper, eggs, shellfish, alcohol, catsup, sauerkraut,
aspirin, tobacco, most drugs, and noodles just to mention a few.  To
correct an overly acidic body I added alkaline foods such as honey,
avocados, corn, most fresh fruits and vegetables, maple syrup, molasses,
raisins, and soy products.  Most fresh fruits and vegetables are

considered alkaline foods. I do add an extra food source or mineral supplement for additional calcium and magnesium. Sweetening with all natural honey can all aid in creating an alkaline body. Following these few action steps listed above resulted in a domino effect, and started healing my body and reversing the aging process.

After discontinuing the junk foods and eating right, I felt better with more energy. Secondly, believing in the higher being is prerequisite to a healthy lifestyle, because it is God's will that we maintain a healthy body. Hence, his will combined with your own will can result in total healing. Just don't give up but keep moving toward perfection, because how can we accomplish anything if we feel tired, depressed, and rundown. Although I cannot predict my longevity, I do still have control over my lifestyle today, which enables me, a woman in her forties, to continue moving toward reawakened goals. I have a fresh outlook on life with renewed creativity as that good old zest haaaas returned!!! But you must stay focused, and keep the body healthy and replenished with proper nutrition.

I could not even think properly or logically reason without these dietary changes. As my past behavior was not by any sense of the word considered reasonable, and did not realize my irrational behavior until my mind and body was free from the chemicals and toxins. I would sleep literally sometimes sleep 10 hours or more and wake up tired. But once toxins were beginning to be eliminated, I started to sleep 5 to 7 hours. One can in fact achieve optimal health, while reversing the premature aging process. Proper dietary habits along with exercise are all essential to a healthy life, as well as proper levels of oxygen contribute to proper circulation and blood flow to the brain. Oxygen is essential to total and complete healing and is achieved through deep breathing. Exercise not only causes increased circulation and blood flow, but oxygen flow as well. Although we focus generally on the fit body, it further includes the whole person and the most important part, the mind. The mind needs to be able to function in order for the other parts of the body to function properly.

Another most important aspect of maintaining health is the gift of knowledge. It is the ultimate factor in our ability to know how to maintain a healthy mind and body.  We must learn and educate ourselves daily, and it is a never-ending process.  Reading not only gives us a healthy outlook on life, but it keeps our mind alert and well.  As I am able to think more logically with a positive view of my life, as I try to read and learn about this broad and beautiful world daily.  Feeling I can contribute just as my ancestors before me to build a better world.  Far more than I could ever imagine in my meager psyche, that I too can and must contribute.  Realizing one person can in fact change the face of a nation and impact the world.  As there have been many individuals before me who made many small and large contributions to make this great land, and I would relish the opportunity to even be considered in this company.  The company of African American Doctor Daniel Hale Williams who founded, Provident Hospital, the nations first interracial hospital in1891, and credited with performing the first successful open heart surgery July 10, 1893.  We must all be proactive and try to obtain the needed test to detect abnormalities before serious illness occur.  Every one should obtain a full body arterial scan which ranges about $120 in price to help detect abnormalities in our arteries prior to experiencing a brain (stroke) or heart attack.  It is well worth the price, if you can save your life by following up with proper treatment.  Most deaths as well as nursing home disabilities are related to circulatory (arterial flow) problems.  The scan results should be taken to a specialist or cardiologist.  Some of the symptoms as previously mentioned for heart problems include tightness of the chest, vomiting, or difficulty breathing.  Stroke symptoms also mentioned include irritability, confusion, weakness, dizziness, difficulty walking, numbness, loss of consciousness, nausea, vomiting, difficulty speaking, drooling and quite often you may return back to normal within a few minutes.  Pain in one part of the body or maybe just a routine headache. This is why it is sometimes termed the silent killer.

Just get checked out and hopefully more than once.  I recommend yearly and followup with immediate treatment as needed and we can reverse the curse with early detection.  I can honestly say since I have changed my view of life through renewing my lifestyle that one can reverse the aging process, and cure many diseases.  I am living proof as I pray to God each day to lead and guide me and take care of me this day. I can even think clearer and reason out important decisions with much more discretion, which reflects more discrete actions. I further have energy like I have not had since, well I can't remember having this kind of energy. I know I have been called and compelled to health and fitness of the mind, body, and soul as I experience much joy in sharing this information through my first love, which is writing.

Being born in poverty as a child I loved to write which probably helped me heal, and deal with somewhat troubling childhood experiences. One might feel as though you are cursed before birth, but through much prayer and perseverance I overcame the adversities. God smiled down on a poor girl from the mean streets of the ghetto, and made a once confused young woman into a new person. I was like a lost sheep that wondered away and lost its direction, but now I'm found and hoping to fulfill my most inevitable predestined future. I have found my way back to some level of sanity through God's sweet mercy and grace. After wrestling with my confused and mostly irresponsible actions in my life, I have finally found peace from the guilt filled past.

This guilt was not just because of my background of being raised in a Christian home, as we feel an enormous responsibility to live upright to be an example for the rest of the world to see. Christians should never make mistakes? But I have found one mistake facilitates additional mistakes, which encompasses even further tumult. I have learned Christianity is from the heart, the inside, and a personal relationship with God. I finally understood God's will of trying to keep us from unnecessary pain by giving us specific guidelines to live by. But he further forgives and still loves us if we make mistakes, and as long as his resoluteness abides with me I will continue in his arms of mercy. God had forgiven me a long time ago, but I had not forgiven myself. Forgiven means to be excused from a fault or offense, or released from an obligation. You are ultimately liberated and free from whatever condition, that may cause you much regret and pain, which is one of the greatest gifts from above. As I have cried and prayed often for forgiveness from God, I remember reading a passage from the Bible, *"Her sins, which are many are forgiven, ....Thy sins are forgiven"*. As I would read over and over but never really fully understanding it or feeling a sense of peace until a few years after the last baby was aborted.

Afterwhich, I was blessed with a call that I felt was from God to care for my ailing mother as eventual catastrophe occurred with her untimely death, I would once again be haunted but would read once more another verse which pressed deeply upon my heart, "*My sheep hear my voice and know them, and they follow me and I give unto them eternal life and they shall never perish, neither shall any man pluck them out of my hand*".

As we come to the realization and understanding our inappropriate behavior, and attempt to change our life we start to understand God's plan and sacrifice of his son Jesus. God knew that as human beings upon this earth with so many immeasurable choices, that in fact we would make mistakes. And even though we may have made some very dreadful mistakes, one of the reasons God gave of his son, Jesus, as an ultimate sacrifice was not only to show us his great love, but for us to grasp the fact that no sin is too big to be forgiven. This is the reason for the ultimate suffering and sacrifice of his son Jesus. Although I may not have forgotten my mistakes, God has removed my mistakes from his record of my life.

God has made each individual unique. This is because no one person can possibly retain all the possible various combinations of knowledge to this vast universe. It is too immense for any one human mind. Hence, God in his infinite wisdom has given each individual their own unique set of information and expertise to combine with others to give completeness to our existence. We all must recognize our calling and fulfill the obligation, not only for ourselves but for the betterment of world. And although we are directly created from moles of our ancestors, we are in fact not our ancestors nor are we an imprecision, but rather a new and evolving culture distinct from any other generation.

I was like a lost sheep and while others may have very differing circumstances, the basic premise of being the lost sheep may be quite similar.  No matter the particular factors encompassing bad decisions, ultimately the domino effect of the lost sheep results in irresponsible and tragic life altering conclusions.  Choices possibly predetermined even before your very existence that may have catapulted into an ultimate choice-less situation.  Also self-inflicted decisions I made that caused me to be forced into yet more bad situations, which can leave you choice-less and your destiny ultimately in the wrongful hands of others.

As I share this information for the lost sheep like myself, a person who may continue to make errors in judgment and wonders why me.  A person who desires change, but may not know how or where to start.  But today the lost sheep can and must take control of their life and make logical decisions based on pass negative experiences, and then move toward the most positive choices through continued education.  This is the most positive choice as we move out of the guilt and shame toward achieving some level of happiness for ourselves, while preparing ourselves as positive role models for the future generations in the process.  We must change our seemingly decaying destiny for a more positive existence.  For past choices in this country as well as one's own personal life choices may not all be perfect, but we must move pass these negative choices and fill it with more positive ones.  We not only have a choice but an obligation to make the right choices for a better life for ourselves, and the world around.  No matter how many bad choices you have made you can overcome your mistakes, just merely start by placing limitations on the unwarranted behavior in your life.  You cannot live a happy and fulfilling life by continuing to adhere to irrational behavior patterns.  We must in fact find the causation factor for this behavior, which can include repercussions from what we choose to eat to whom we will choose to befriend.  You have a choice and you must choose a life to make a significant difference not only in your life, but in other lives as well.  Making the right choices encompasses placing some behavioral limits in your life.

While placing limits in your life can prove rather difficult, one simply should just keep trying to achieve that perfection you once may have known or dreamed of and eventually a new and brighter day will emerge. Always continuing to remember, it is never too late. I will never forget my first year in college how I had the honor of sharing the classroom with a sixty-year young lady, who was working toward her teaching certificate. As one person trying to make a difference, I truly believe one person can change the world. Just as Moses, Jesus, Abe, MLK, and countless others, we must strive to be remembered in this world by our good works. Because in the end beauty passes, but finding yourself and having the fulfillment of living a good life is not only memorable but results in peace of mind.

No matter what you feel you may have done, and what mistakes you may make, everything happens for a reason. God has left you upon this earth for a reason, and though you may constantly come against many foes you shall continue to be steadfast and strong because the Lord has something great for you to do. He needs you because you will help save some lives, clothe and feed the hungry. You are God's pride and joy and as you appear to constantly battle just to survive on a daily basis, it is only because of whom you are and you are a significant and vital part of God's plan. Do not give up it will get better! God is getting you ready for his plan for your life.

*As I wish all of you much peace, love, and prosperity. May we all share God's never ending wisdom and guidance residing in us as we move toward greater heights, for we were all once one of the lost sheep.*

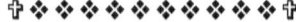

*"I am come that they may have life and have it more abundantly.*
*St John*